After four years and ten cycles of treatment, Jacqueline Tomlins has learned a lot about infertility—not just the nitty-gritty of hormones and sperm, but how to take control of treatment rather than letting it take control of you.

Jacqueline Tomlins has worked as a teacher, researcher, trainer and advocate and is now a full-time writer. Her travel book *A Girl's Own Adventure: Across Africa Any Way Any How* was published recently. She has also written about infertility for a number of newspapers and journals.

The Infertility Handbook

A guide to making babies

Jacqueline Tomlins

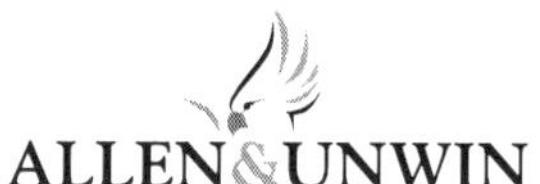

First published in 2003

Allen & Unwin
83 Alexander Street
Crows Nest NSW 2065
Australia
Phone: (61 2) 8425 0100
Fax: (61 2) 9906 2218
Email: info@allenandunwin.com
Web: www.allenandunwin.com

National Library of Australia
Cataloguing-in-Publication entry:

Tomlins, Jacqueline Ruth.
The infertility handbook : a guide to making babies.

Bibliography.
Includes index.
ISBN 1 74114 145 1.

1. Infertility—Treatment—Popular works. 2. Human reproductive technology—Popular works. 3. Fertilization in vitro, Human—Popular works. I. Title.

618.17806

Set in 11/14 pt Granjon by Bookhouse, Sydney
Printed by McPhersons Printing Group, Maryborough, Victoria

10 9 8 7 6 5 4 3 2 1

For Corin
and everyone who helped create him

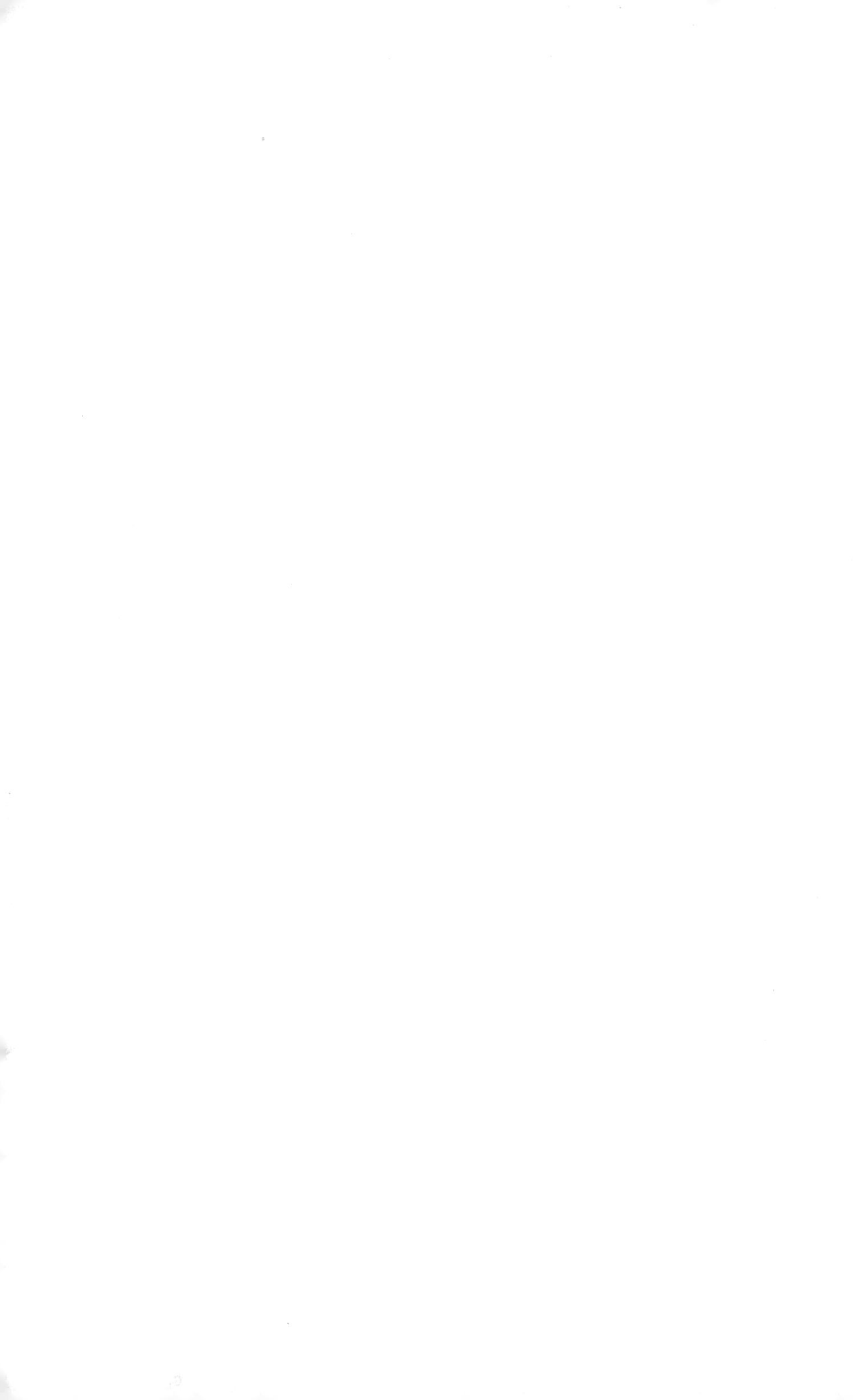

Contents

Foreword

When I first met Jacqui, I remember being particularly impressed by her knowledge and understanding of the scientific, and not so scientific, aspects of infertility and its treatment. I was also amazed by her ability to articulate the roller-coaster of emotions and frustrations experienced by infertility patients. Throughout her long journey with infertility, Jacqui managed to develop strategies and coping mechanisms that helped her retain perspective, and continue to be optimistic and enthusiastic about her ongoing treatment. Thank goodness she decided to write this book!

As infertility specialists, we struggle to help our patients understand their infertility and to make informed decisions about management and we cross our fingers and hope that we are doing a good enough job. But I feel sure that, well-intentioned as we are, there are always some gaps left. There is no doubt that being well-informed and having a sound understanding of the issues empowers patients and their partners to feel more in control of their condition, to make rational management choices and to be realistic about possible outcomes.

Until now, there have been very few resources which provide medical and scientific information in a practical format which is both easy to understand and relevant to the Australian population. *The Infertility Handbook* is extremely well-researched, factual, comprehensive, up-to-date and inclusive of the full range of available treatments.

But, perhaps most importantly, it offers sage, valuable and sensible advice about how to cope with the many and varied emotions that come with infertility. *The Infertility Handbook* should be read and kept by the bedside for continuing reference by everyone who suffers from infertility, and by their families and friends. It is written in a spirit of generosity with the aim of improving the experiences of other patients and their families. *The Infertility Handbook* is a unique, profound and valuable contribution to the management of infertility.

Dr Catharyn J Stern
MBBS FRANZCOG, MRCOG, CREI,
Gynaecologist, Infertility Specialist and Reproductive
Endocrinologist, Melbourne IVF and Royal Women's Hospital

September 2003

Acknowledgements

This book could not have been written without the support of a number of people. First and foremost, my thanks to Dr Kate Stern from Melbourne IVF who had the idea in the first place, who indulged all my nit-picking questions, who carefully checked my drafts to ensure complete accuracy and who lent her full support throughout. Jenny Blood, Senior Counsellor, Melbourne IVF gave generously of her time and patience in reading all the drafts. This book, particularly the latter chapters, benefits from her enormous understanding and experience. Donna Ramselaar, Nursing Team Leader, and Suzanne Lemaire, Nurse Educator at Melbourne IVF, were both indispensable in ensuring the details of all the treatment protocols were accurate and up to date and that I had covered everything. Thank you both for your thoughtfulness and attention to detail.

Dr Ruth McNair, Senior Lecturer, Director of Undergraduate Studies, Department of General Practice at The University of Melbourne provided expert advice for Chapter 7, 'Single Women and Lesbian Couples—Options for Conceiving'. Kristen Walker,

Senior Lecturer, Faculty of Law at the University of Melbourne helped to shed light on the complex legal situation around access to infertility treatment for single women and lesbians. Thanks also to Judy Small, Associate at Slater & Gordon Lawyers.

Sandra Dill, Executive Director of ACCESS Australia Infertility Network read the manuscript and arranged for a number of people to provide feedback. Thanks to Sandra, Leanne Marsh, Bronwyn Cantrill and Dr Steve Sonneveld. Dr Kim Matthews at IVF Australia, also read and checked the manuscript. Dr David Edgar, Scientific Director at Melbourne IVF generously provided photographs.

My good friends Lee FitzRoy and Nicole Hayes talked with me on many occasions about the book as it developed, read drafts and provided useful and detailed feedback. Thanks girls.

I wanted this book to reflect the experiences of people who had, in whatever way, faced challenges in creating the family they wanted. Many people agreed to tell me their stories and allowed me to share them with others by putting them in this book. They told me their stories with openness, honesty and integrity, even when it was clearly very difficult and painful for them to do so. What they did was, I believe, an act of courage. This book—and, I hope, its readers—benefits from those acts of courage. My sincerest thanks to Andrew and Andrea, Darcy, Greg and Tracy, Hannah and Charles, Jacki and Maria, Kris and Miranda, Lee, Mark, Tanya and Wendy.

Finally, special thanks to Sarah who shared this journey with me—both the infertility and the book about it—who supported me while I wrote and who offered tea and encouragement whenever I flagged. Thankfully, she was way too busy with our baby to read any drafts.

Introduction

Most people grow up believing that having children is a normal and natural part of life. We take for granted that, when the time is right, we'll be able to create the family we want. We don't expect it will be difficult. We don't expect we'll need anyone else's help. For some people, though, creating a family turns out to be a bit more complicated. If you've picked up this book, you're probably one of them.

Perhaps, even though you have been trying for a while, you haven't conceived, and that little niggling doubt you developed a few months ago is starting to turn into a quiet but constant worry. Perhaps you're wondering if there's something wrong with you—or your partner—and whether there's a treatment out there that might help. Perhaps you know already you're going to need some kind of medical intervention to get or stay pregnant. Whatever your circumstances, this book is intended to help you find your way through the often complex and confusing world of infertility and its treatments.

It may be you don't actually have a fertility problem—it's just taking you a bit longer to conceive and, in time, it will resolve itself. It may be you have a condition that is quite common and easily remedied that's affecting your fertility. It may be you have something more significant wrong, which requires complex treatment, including the various forms of in vitro fertilisation (IVF). Sometimes—quite often, in fact—infertility is *unexplained* and treatment can involve a bit of trial and error. Sometimes, all the medical science in the world won't help you make a baby.

Not everyone who has a fertility problem will seek medical help, and many people will choose *not* to go down the IVF track. This book is primarily for people who *are* thinking about getting some form of medical assistance to help them make a baby, and for others who, for various reasons, may need assistance to help them conceive.

If you do end up having any kind of treatment, you will be embarking on a journey, a journey that might be short and smooth or long and bumpy. You will find yourselves exploring unfamiliar territory and facing all sorts of new challenges. There will be ups and downs along the way, times when things are more or less difficult, times when you get tired and need to take a break. As with any journey, it can help to know what lies ahead, to have a map of all the different routes so you know where each might take you. It can help to have a guide to answer questions, to explain things along the way. *The Infertility Handbook* is such a guide for your infertility journey.

How you use this guide will depend on your particular circumstances and where you are on this journey. You may want to get a general idea of what to expect before you even see a specialist, or before you decide to have any treatment. If you do have treatment, you might use the guide to clarify the protocol you are on, to look up the terminology, to find out about a procedure, to check what comes next. At any stage, you might want to read about how other people dealt with a situation. You might also want to share this guide with friends or family so they have an idea of what you're going through.

The guide begins by describing what happens when you first approach your GP with an infertility problem. It then looks at what happens if you are referred to an infertility specialist. It outlines the factors that might be contributing to your problem and takes you, step by step, through the various medical options available. It also explores the personal and emotional implications of dealing with all this.

Infertility raises questions that go to the core of who we are: questions about identity, about our roles in families and relationships, about our life choices. What can make infertility treatment tough is that, at the very time we are having to deal with these huge personal issues, we are faced with what, for many of us, is the first, and the most significant, medical treatment we've ever had to undergo.

For the purpose of this book I have tried to separate the physical and emotional aspects of treatment—not something you can do when you're actually going through the process. Some days you will want information, facts that are clear, concise and accurate. You may have forgotten to ask your doctor something. You may have left the surgery more confused than when you went in. You will want answers. On other days you might need emotional support, maybe after a negative result, a cancelled cycle, or just a bad day. Every now and again, you'll need reassurance that your experience is completely normal and, like others before you, you'll get through.

The more you know about infertility and its treatment, the more able you will be to manage it successfully. One of the common experiences of undergoing any treatment—particularly IVF—is a sense of powerlessness, a feeling your life has been overtaken, that you no longer have control. Being well informed and actively participating in decisions about your treatment are ways of taking back some of that control. In my experience—and that of many other people with fertility problems—understanding the complexities of the process goes a long way to getting through it successfully.

After almost five years and ten IVF cycles, I've learnt a lot about infertility and its treatment; not just the nitty-gritty of hormones and sperm, but about the way in which it can affect your life and—if you let it—how it can overwhelm you. Infertility treatment is tough—there's no doubt about that—but there are things you can do to make it easier. If I were starting again, I would try to manage my treatment in the same way as I manage my work or any other major part of my life. I'd pay it careful attention. I'd prioritise it, plan for it, reassess and review it. I'd give it space and time, not just try to squeeze it into an already full schedule. As far as possible—and this isn't always easy—I'd try to maintain a balance, try not to let it take over my life.

One of the constant complaints by people dealing with infertility is the lack of understanding of others—not just friends, family, or colleagues, but politicians, media commentators and religious leaders. Sometimes, wherever we look we are confronted with people who just don't get it. That is why so many of us share this journey only with our partners or most intimate friends.

This book is written by someone who has also taken the journey and is filled with the stories of many others with whom we share the path. My aim in writing it is to provide support in some small way for your journey—the way other people helped me through mine. I will resist the temptation to wish you good luck—though that certainly plays a part—and instead wish you three things I hope will help: patience, fortitude and a sense of humour.

> It was definitely worth doing the infertility treatment. It's hard and it's lonely, but it's worth a go. If we hadn't done it, we would always have regretted it. It's the best thing we ever did, and we're thankful that we were in a position where we could afford it and that the technology was there. Tracy's Dad still calls our son 'Miracle Boy'.
>
> Greg, partner of Tracy, father of Oscar

1

It's just not working

Exploring problems with conception

If you have been having unprotected sex with your partner for some time and have not conceived, you might be starting to wonder why. Most people, once they stop using contraception, imagine they will fall pregnant pretty quickly. In fact, it's not uncommon to start worrying pretty soon after you start trying. It's important to remember, however, that normal fertility is regarded as achieving a pregnancy within two years of regular sex—much longer than most people think. Unless you have a specific, pre-existing problem of which you are aware—painful or irregular periods, previous surgery, prior chemotherapy or other relevant treatment, or if the woman is over 35—it is probably not worth seeking specialist help until you have been trying to conceive for at least 12 months. Statistics show that approximately 80 per cent of couples who will ultimately conceive, do so in the first 12 months of having regular, unprotected intercourse.

To a certain extent, this will depend on whether you have been having sex at the time when you are most fertile (at ovulation) which happens around the middle of your menstrual cycle. If you are having regular sex, say two to three times a week, it is likely to be coinciding with ovulation anyway. If you want to be sure, it is possible to monitor your ovulation at home by yourself (see 'Monitoring your ovulation') and time your intercourse to coincide. Lots of couples do this if they have been trying for a little while to get pregnant without success. It can be a good way of doing something proactive, and it is relatively easy and private. Timed intercourse can, however, get a bit stressful, and it might not be something you want to do for a long time. Many couples find the lack of spontaneity makes it awkward or difficult and the pressure to perform at a specific time takes the pleasure and intimacy out of sex.

Monitoring your ovulation

In a normal 28-day cycle ovulation should occur around day 14. If your cycle is shorter (up to 26 days) or longer (up to 32 days) you may ovulate anywhere between day 11 and day 17. The second half of your cycle is more or less constant—that means you ovulate approximately 14 days before your period, irrespective of the length of your cycle. The problem is, however, that you might ovulate on day 14 one month, then on day 16 the next, and on day 15 the one after that. Some women are very regular and consistent and some are not. There are three basic ways of monitoring your ovulation at home: tracking your *basal body temperature*, checking your vaginal mucus and using a urine testing kit.

Monitoring your basal body temperature

Your basal body temperature (BBT) changes at different stages during your cycle. By noting these changes you can track the course of your cycle. You cannot, however, *predict* when you will ovulate,

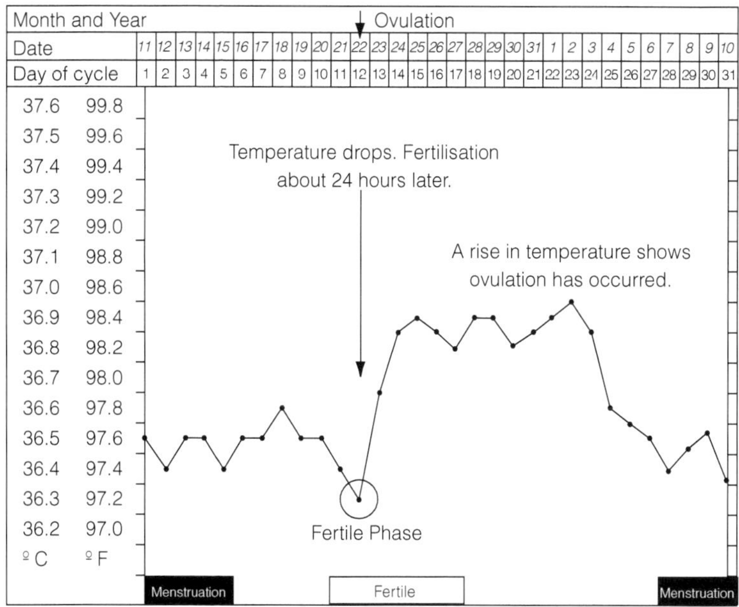

Chart for tracking basal body temperature

you can only work out that ovulation has occurred *after* it has happened. The idea is to track your temperature for a few months so you might begin to see a pattern. Keeping track of your BBT can help you get in tune with your cycle, though it can become a bit of a nuisance after a while—just another daily reminder that something's not quite right. If you do try it, it might be best to limit it to, say, three or four months.

You will need to buy a special BBT thermometer from your chemist—an ordinary mercury thermometer, or one used for fevers, is not calibrated enough. You will also need to draw up a chart like the one above and keep it by your bedside with your thermometer. On day 1, the first day of your period, take your temperature first thing in the morning, before you get out of bed—even before you have wandered down the hallway to the bathroom, or had a cup of tea. For the best accuracy, you should place the thermometer in the

> You know you are ovulating, then you have to somehow communicate this to your partner. You either make a decision to make love, or you have to subtly try to indicate that maybe it's a good idea, or you might decide to seduce him, or you just have to be really blunt and say, 'By the way, I'M OVULATING!', which isn't very conducive to love-making. It's really difficult. You might not feel like making love and it changes the purpose of being together. He feels like he has to perform and thinks, 'You only want me for my sperm'. You can't really say, 'Yes, that's exactly why I want you!'.
>
> Lee

vagina, but lots of women place it under the tongue instead. Mark your temperature on the corresponding day on your chart.

If you are ovulating normally your body temperature should drop on the day of ovulation and then rise by 0.5 to 1.0 degree Celsius immediately afterwards. The rise in temperature is caused by the increased production of progesterone. Your most fertile time is from one day before your temperature drops until one day after it is elevated.

> I was keeping track of my cycle, doing the basal body temperature thing. It was really complicated. One month I was going up to Canberra for a conference and I ovulated that weekend, so I got Mark to fly up to Canberra. I'm sure this is difficult for lots of couples trying to conceive while also trying to maintain an intimate relationship with your lover.
>
> Lee

Checking your vaginal mucus

Most women develop a slippery vaginal mucus a few days prior to ovulation. Some women are very aware of this and some barely notice it. Over the course of a few menstrual cycles you can monitor your mucus, making a note of what day in your cycle it appears, how long it lasts and whether the amount of mucus increases over time. The mucus reaches its peak on the day of your ovulation. You may be able to distinguish this quite clearly, or it might just be a little vague. This method can be effective, and can be a good alternative to monitoring your temperature, but it doesn't work for everybody.

Using a urine testing kit

It is possible to buy an ovulation testing kit over the counter at your local chemist. The kit contains a number of small plastic units onto which you place drops of urine with a small pipette. The units measure your level of *luteinising hormone* (LH) (see Chapter 3), which rises immediately before you ovulate. If the test identifies a raised level of LH (your 'LH surge') a line will appear on the unit. You ovulate approximately 24 to 36 hours after the surge.

This is probably an easier and more accurate way of determining your ovulation than using the basal body temperature or vaginal mucus methods. Using the kit can be useful for one cycle if your cycles are basically regular, but if your cycles vary by more than five days you may need to monitor your ovulation over a long period of time, which can become very expensive. For cost reasons it is not really a practical way of tracking your ovulation over a long period of time. Some hospitals do provide a urine testing service where you drop off a urine sample in the morning, and call later in the day to find out the result. Check with your clinic or local hospital for details.

Seeing your GP

If you have been having sex regularly around your fertile time for a year or so and still haven't conceived, you might want to take that first step. For most people this will mean talking to your family doctor or local GP, though some people go straight to a gynaecologist. Some people also seek advice from a naturopath, Chinese herbalist or other alternative health practitioner before, or as well as, seeing a western medical specialist. The extent to which these various practitioners will investigate your problem will vary enormously.

Alternative practitioners may focus on your diet, lifestyle, stress levels, and overall general health, and may prescribe a range of natural or herbal remedies that may or may not help. Some GPs will refer you immediately to an infertility specialist without doing any investigations themselves. Other GPs, and most gynaecologists, will do a few preliminary investigations. This may involve asking general questions about your sexual and medical history and doing a broad health check of both partners. At this early stage there are some routine tests you can have done.

Women may have a:

- pap smear to check for any abnormal cervical cells
- breast examination to check for lumps and general health.
- blood test for Rubella (German measles)—rubella can cause developmental abnormalities during pregnancy and, even if you think you have been vaccinated as a child, your immunity may be low and you may need to be re-vaccinated
- blood test in the second half of your menstrual cycle to check your progesterone levels—progesterone is a key hormone that plays an important part in reproduction.

In some cases, a blood test for hepatitis B and C, and HIV will also be performed.

Men may have a semen analysis to assess the health of their sperm (see below). Semen analysis is a highly specialised procedure and it is worth asking your doctor to send the sample to a specialist, rather than a local laboratory. Even if you have an analysis done at this stage, any infertility specialist you see later will repeat the test again later. In some cases, a test for hepatitis B and C, and HIV will also be performed.

Seeing an infertility specialist

As a result of these initial investigations, you may discover the cause of your problem and be able to resolve it easily or, in the course of doing them, you may fall pregnant naturally. If not, your next step is to ask for a referral to an infertility specialist. If you live in a major urban area you will have a choice of specialists and clinics; if you live in the country you probably will not. The bigger clinics have a number of doctors from whom you can choose, and some have satellite clinics in outlying areas. Smaller, regional practices are more likely to have just one or two specialists. (All currently accredited clinics in Australia are listed in 'Information and resources' at the back of the book.) There are a number of ways you can find out more about the different clinics and their doctors:

- check the clinic website—most give short biographies of the specialists and an overview of their philosophy and treatment
- ask the clinic to send out any information—most clinics have a 'Guide for patients' or something similar; they may also have a video that introduces the clinic and outlines treatment
- phone the clinic and ask to speak to someone who has time to answer some general questions. You can always start with the nursing, administrative staff, or counsellors rather than a doctor, if you prefer
- find out if the clinic runs evening information sessions and go along to one
- arrange to speak to a clinic counsellor, either over the phone or in person
- talk to someone who has had treatment at that clinic
- find out if there is a support group associated with the clinic and call them, or contact one of the national infertility organisations
- make an appointment with a doctor, and ask some preliminary questions; if you do not feel comfortable with them, try a different doctor.

In general, this field of medicine is highly regulated and, in Australia, all clinics have to be accredited by a professional regulating body established by the Fertility Society of Australia. You can be reasonably assured, therefore, that all the clinics are operating to a high minimum standard. This is not to say, however, that they don't vary. The bigger clinics will have access to greater facilities and a broader range of expertise. Some practitioners will be more experienced than others; some will stick to tried and tested practices, while their colleagues will be more inclined to try new, 'cutting-edge' or experimental protocols. You will find the majority of specialists in the field are men, but there are a number of women. Most people tend to go with their gut feeling when choosing a doctor or a clinic; the person on the end of the phone is friendly and helpful, or someone knows someone who says Dr Bloggs is good.

The first consultation

When you have decided who you want to see, ring and make an appointment. Like any specialist there may be a few weeks' or even months' wait. Your first consultation will more than likely be a discussion. You may be asked to fill out a form with some preliminary questions while you are waiting to see the doctor. The specialist will then ask a lot of questions as he or she tries to get a broad, general understanding of your particular circumstances. They may or may not perform a physical examination—more often this is planned for a later session.

The doctor will take a detailed medical history of both partners. There is roughly an equal chance of a male, female or combined factor contributing to the infertility (where the cause is known); that is, in about a third of cases, there is something wrong with the woman, in another third there is something wrong with the man, and in another third there is something about the combination of the two that causes the problem. The aim at this stage is to do a thorough clinical evaluation to identify any apparent reasons why you aren't conceiving.

Listed below is the range of questions you can expect to be asked. You may like to jot down notes about these questions so you have your answers clear in your mind when you are speaking with your doctor. The questions may not be asked in this order, and your doctor may focus more on one area than another, depending on your particular circumstances. Some may not be asked at all. You may find some of the questions embarrassing or intrusive; you really just have to take a deep breath and answer them as fully and honestly as possible. There are no right or wrong answers and if you can't answer them all, or if you are unclear on some of the details, don't worry.

For the woman

Sexual history

- Have you been having regular sex? (NB: Men and women sometimes differ on their definition of 'regular sex.')
- How much attention have you paid to the timing of that sex—that is, have you been having sex at the time of ovulation?
- Are there any problems having sex?
- Is it painful or difficult in any way?
- What methods of birth control have you used?
- Have you ever been fitted with an interuterine contraceptive device (IUD or IUCD) or had an injection of Depo Provera?
- Have you ever had—or do you have now—a sexually transmitted disease; for example, herpes, chlamydia, syphilis or gonorrhoea?

Your menstrual cycle

- How long is your cycle—28/30/32 days?
- Are your periods regular?

- Do you have symptoms of ovulation—changes in vaginal mucus, pelvic pain in the middle of your cycle, or a temperature rise in the second phase of your cycle?
- Have you ever had pre-menstrual spotting, abnormal bleeding, painful periods, vaginal discharge, general pelvic pain or discomfort?

Your gynaecological history

- Have you had any previous pregnancies, miscarriages, ectopic pregnancies, caesareans, successful births or terminations?
- If so, were there any particular problems with these?
- Is there any chance you may have had an infection?
- Have you ever been identified as having an 'incompetent' cervix, or any abnormalities of the cervix?

Your medical history

- Do you have any current medical illnesses?
- Are you taking any medications for an existing medical condition?
- Do you suffer from diabetes?
- Have you had any pelvic or abdominal surgery or anything that may have resulted in infection—for example, a ruptured appendix or cyst or a bowel injury?
- Have you had any other surgical procedures or operations in the past?
- Have you ever had chemotherapy or radiation treatment?

Your family history and lifestyle

- Is there any family history of infertility or problems with hormones or periods?
- Are there any genetic disorders or illnesses in the family?
- Do you smoke, and if so, how much?
- Do you drink a lot of coffee or tea?
- Do you use any non-prescription or recreational drugs?

- What's your diet like?
- How are your stress levels?
- Where do you work?
- What is your occupation?

Your doctor will also make an assessment of your general appearance, including your weight and facial hair. A low body weight may be associated with *anovulation* (not ovulating) (see Chapter 3), and increased body weight may also be associated with anovulation and with *polycystic ovarian syndrome* (PCOS) (see Chapter 3). One symptom of PCOS is more than usual facial hair growth. They may also check your general cardiovascular health—heart and blood pressure—and respiratory system. In some instances a doctor may do a short vaginal examination, examining your uterus with his or her fingers (the old fashioned 'internal').

For the man

Sexual history

- Have you been having regular sex?
- How much attention have you paid to the timing of that sex?
- Are there any problems having sex?
- Is it painful in any way?
- Do you have any difficulties achieving an erection, having an orgasm or ejaculating?

- Have you had any children previously, or are you aware of any previous pregnancies?
- Have you ever had—or do you now have—a sexually transmitted disease; for example, herpes, chlamydia, syphilis or gonorrhoea?
- Have you ever had a vasectomy or a reversal of a vasectomy?

Your medical history

- Have you had any operations or illnesses around the pelvic or abdominal area—hernia operation or surgery on the scrotum, for example, or bladder neck surgery?
- Have you ever had any sports injuries to the groin that may have resulted in testicular trauma?
- Have you ever suffered from any kind of inflammation of the testes, sore or tender testes, or have you ever experienced a torsion (twisting) of the testes?
- Did you have undescended testes—*cryptorchidism*—as a baby? If so, when was this diagnosed and treated?
- Did you have any medical illnesses, particularly mumps as a child or adolescent?
- Have you ever taken medication for inflammatory bowel disease or blood pressure?
- Are you currently on any medication?
- Have you experienced any kind of viral infection or fever in the last six months?
- Do you have diabetes or thyroid problems?
- Have you ever had chemotherapy or radiation treatment?

Your family history and lifestyle

- Is there a family history of infertility or other related problems?
- Are there any genetic disorders or illnesses in the family?
- What is your occupation?

- Do you work with pesticides, plastics, solvents, paints or other chemical materials or radiation?
- Do you regularly use saunas or hot tubs, or do anything that might result in an increase in the temperature of your testes—for example, regular, long-distance driving?
- Do you smoke, and if so, how much?
- Do you use recreational drugs, such as marijuana?

Five weeks after we were married, Andrew was diagnosed with testicular cancer, which meant he was going to have to have chemotherapy. So we decided to freeze sperm because we knew we wouldn't be able to conceive naturally afterwards. He had three months of chemotherapy and after he finished that, after he recovered, we pretty much started IVF straightaway.

Andrea

Your doctor will process all this information and attempt to determine if there is anything immediately identifiable as the cause of your problem. More than likely, however, they will tell you they need to do further investigations. It is perhaps worth noting here that between 20 to 25 per cent of couples who present for infertility treatment are diagnosed with *idiopathic* (or unexplained) *infertility*—that is, after investigation the cause remains unexplained. This doesn't mean you can't be treated, only that the exact cause of your problem is not diagnosable.

Finding a specific cause for the problem can sometimes actually be a relief, especially if that cause can be treated. Sometimes, not finding a cause—being told everything appears completely normal—can be more frustrating. I know, for me, constantly being told that everything was functioning normally, and that there was no explanation for my failure to conceive was very difficult at times.

The physical examination

The second part of your clinical assessment is the physical examination. If your doctor doesn't perform this at your first consultation, a time will be arranged to do it pretty soon afterwards. Most people find these a bit embarrassing, but they shouldn't hurt, and they don't take long. For the woman, it will usually be done just before ovulation—around the middle of your cycle if you are ovulating normally. If you are not ovulating, it can be done at any time. For the man, it can be done at any time. You have the right to have another person present with you during any physical examination, either your partner, or a nurse.

For the woman

Examination of the woman is most often done by a transvaginal pelvic ultrasound, a commonly used procedure for assessing the overall health of your internal reproductive system. The transvaginal pelvic ultrasound is usually—and somewhat deceptively—referred to as a 'scan'. You would not be the first woman in the world to picture one of those unobtrusive procedures you have seen on the telly where a doctor rubs gel onto your belly and gently moves a probe across your tummy. That's not what we're talking about here: the transvaginal scan is *internal*. It involves a probe being gently inserted into your vagina.

You will be shown into a room and asked to remove your clothes from the waist down, including your underwear. Often the doctor leaves the room while you do this, or at least stands behind a screen. You then step up onto a special chair that has moveable rests for your legs, and you cover your lower half with a sheet. The doctor will take the probe and cover it with either a condom, one finger of a latex glove, or—and I kid you not—cling wrap, and squirt lubricant onto the top. He or she might ask you to shuffle down a little, open your legs and, with those famous words, 'just relax', will slide the probe into your vagina.

Your uterus will appear on the screen, though you might not recognise it at first, and can be forgiven for thinking it bears a remarkable similarity to the Milky Way on a clear night. Your doctor should explain exactly what he or she is looking at. If there is anything that is unclear or that you don't understand, *ask*. They should show you how to identify your ovaries and the follicles that contains your eggs—they look a bit like a small bunch of grapes—and you may also be able to see the lining of your uterus, which is easier to identify when it is thick.

Your doctor will see a whole lot more than this. They will use the scan to check that your uterus is in the right position, is the normal size, and that there are no congenital abnormalities—things you are born with that aren't quite right (see Chapter 4). They will check for the presence of fibroids, tumours, endometrial polpys or polycystic ovaries (see Chapter 3), all of them things that can affect your fertility. They will measure and assess the thickness of the lining of your uterus and whether this is normal for the phase of your cycle. They will check that your ovaries look normal and note whether there are any follicles—the sacs that contain your eggs—developing; sometimes they will be able to see one ovary more clearly than the other. They will also look at your fallopian tubes and check for *hydrosalpinges* (blockages) (see Chapter 3).

For the man

The examination of the man may be performed by your doctor, or you may be referred to an *andrologist*, a specialist in men's fertility. They will examine your external reproductive organs, checking your penis, the size and firmness of your testes and whether you have *varicoceles*—small varicose veins on the testes which can affect fertility (see Chapter 3). They will also evaluate the possibility of any blockages or obstructions in the internal ducts through which your semen travels.

A more comprehensive evaluation performed by an andrologist may include a general examination of the abdomen and groin region, and a broad check of the neck and chest area to look for any associated illnesses. They will also check the tubular structures of the reproductive organs, the vas deferens and the epididymus, for cysts, swellings or possible obstruction. The examination should not take long and should not be painful.

Standard preliminary tests

It is likely your specialist will propose two preliminary tests as part of this early clinical evaluation irrespective of whether you had them done with your GP: the progesterone test for the woman, normally referred to as a *mid-luteal serum progesterone*, and the semen analysis for the man. At this stage, your specialist is trying to build up a broad picture of your particular circumstances by getting as much information as possible.

Progesterone test

For the progesterone test you will be required to give a blood sample on around day 21 of your cycle—though this will vary depending on the length of your cycle. In order to get an accurate reading of your progesterone levels the test needs to be done in the mid-luteal phase; that is, seven days before your next period. If you are ovulating normally your levels should be high at this stage; a low level may indicate a problem with ovulation. Your doctor will add the results of this test to the rest of the information they have to get a more complete picture of your menstrual cycle.

Semen analysis

A semen analysis can determine whether there is anything wrong with your sperm which may be affecting your fertility. Most clinics

> I think we've been really lucky, though, because you read a lot of books and talk to the counsellors and they always say people feel like they are a failure. We have never felt that way. I don't know if it's because we've been more pragmatic in approaching it all. For us, it's just a medical problem.
>
> Charles

prefer you to produce a sample on site at their infertility laboratory—although there are alternatives (see below). Producing a sample has become popular subject material for comedians and movie makers, but most men find this part of the process a bit awkward and embarrassing. It is certainly one of those occasions when it's helpful to relax—if that's at all possible—and to have your sense of humour close by.

Usually, you will be required to attend the lab at a specified time. When you make your appointment you will be told how to prepare for the test. You should not have had intercourse or ejaculated for at least two, but not more than five, days before giving your sample. You will be given a sterile jar and shown into a private room where you will be asked to produce your sample by masturbation. You cannot use any kind of lubricant. There may be magazines in the room, or sometimes a video to help you. Some clinics may even offer you a drink. You may ask your wife or partner to accompany you. It is important to ensure that all the *ejaculate* makes it into the jar, and it is especially important that the first part gets in as this generally has the highest concentration of sperm. Some clinics might occasionally ask you to produce a split ejaculate, which involves getting semen into two different jars.

It is completely normal to feel anxious and a bit pressured. If it really isn't a happening thing, you can arrange another appointment for a different time. If you think it's just not going to work at all, you can arrange to produce the sample at home so long as you can be sure you can get it to the lab within one to two hours. A delay of more than this will affect the accuracy of the analysis. If you do produce the sample at home you should carry it to the clinic in a pocket to keep it warm.

If you do not feel comfortable producing a sample by masturbation, you can ask the clinic to supply you with a special condom to use during intercourse. Normal condoms cannot be used as most are toxic to sperm. Clinics generally prefer, however, not to use this method as the sample can become contaminated with other cells.

Your specialist may recommend doing a second test eight weeks or so after the first if any abnormalities show up. It is possible for a second test to show different results. This can occur because of the inherent variability of the semen, or because of slight differences in the collection of the sample. If you have had a viral infection up to three months before you produce the sample—a bout of 'flu for example—your sperm may show some abnormalities that could be resolved by the time you do a second test.

The fluid you produce when you ejaculate is referred to as semen. Your sperm is only a small part of that semen—in fact, the sperm cells make up only about 1 per cent. Your sample will be examined under a microscope by a laboratory technician who will assess the following:

- **volume**—the total amount of ejaculate produced (the normal amount is approximately two millilitres, although the quantity is not the most important factor. The medical term for producing no semen is *aspermia.*)
- **concentration**—the number of sperm (both alive and dead) that are in the ejaculate (the normal amount is 20 million sperm per millilitre or more. The medical term for producing no sperm is *azoospermia*, and for few sperm is *oligozoospermia.*)
- **motility**—the number of moving sperm in the ejaculate (the normal amount is about 50 per cent or more, with at least half of those having good forward movement. The medical term for weak or slow moving sperm is *asthenozoospermia.*)
- **velocity**—the average speed at which the sperm travels (the normal speed is 30 microns per second or more).

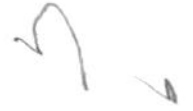

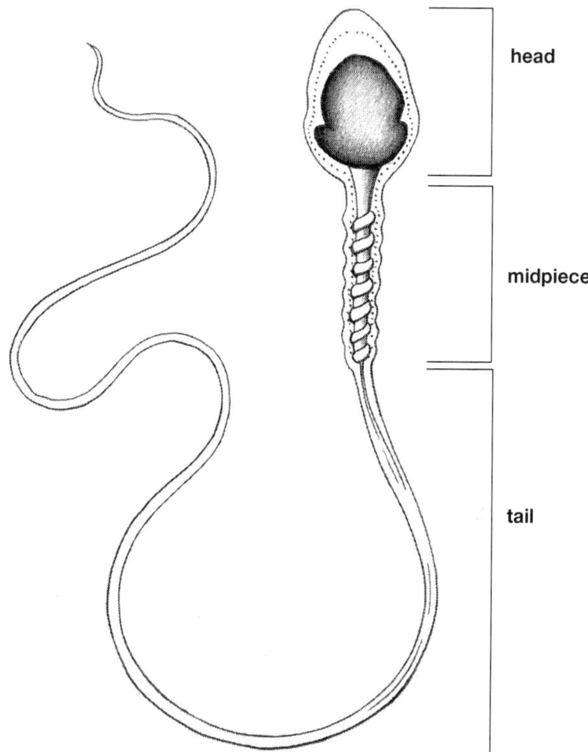

A healthy sperm

- **morphology**—the number of sperm of normal size and shape in the ejaculate (the normal amount is about 15 per cent. The medical term for malformed sperm is *tetraozoospermia*).

Immunobead test

An *immunobead test* is usually carried out at the same time as the semen analysis. This test determines whether or not *anti-sperm antibodies* are present in the semen. These anitbodies attach themselves to the head or tail of the sperm and, where there are sufficient numbers, can make it difficult for the sperm to penetrate the egg. Where sperm antibodies are a problem, your doctor may suggest in vitro fertilisation (IVF) (see Chapter 4).

Further investigations

Your specialist may also suggest a number of further investigations. Which of these they do, and when exactly they do them, will depend on your particular circumstances. Further investigations may include:

- testing the levels of other significant hormones: *follicle stimulating hormone* (FSH), *luteinising hormone* (LH), *thyroid stimulating hormone* (TSH), *androgens* and *prolactin*
- doing a sperm–mucus penetration test (*Kremer test*)
- doing a *postcoital test* (although this is rarely done these days)
- performing a *hysterosalpingogram* (HSG) or a *sonohysterogram* (SonoHSG)
- performing a *laparoscopy* or *hysteroscopy*.

Hormone tests

For the hormone tests, the woman will be required to give a blood sample at a specific time in her cycle. The blood is then analysed to see if she is producing the appropriate levels of the various hormones:

- follicle stimulating hormone (FSH)—responsible for stimulating your ovaries to make the follicles grow
- luteinising hormone (LH)—responsible for ovulation (the release of eggs from the follicle)
- thyroid stimulating hormone (TSH)—activates the thyroid gland (an under or over active thyroid can affect the menstrual cycle)
- prolactin—responsible for stimulating milk production in the breasts (high levels can affect ovulation and the maturation of eggs)
- androgens—the male sex hormones also produced by women in lesser quantities (a high level can affect the development and release of the eggs).

Kremer test

The *Kremer test* examines the capacity of the sperm to penetrate or swim through the mucus that is secreted in the woman's vagina around the time of ovulation. The man will be required to provide a sperm sample, and a swab will be taken of the woman's vaginal mucus at mid cycle. The interaction of the sperm and mucus is then examined under a microscope and analysed using donor sperm and mucus as a controlled comparison. This test is particularly important if the man has been identified as having antisperm antibodies. It will help the doctor evaluate the significance of the presence of those antibodies.

Postcoital test

A similar, less accurate test is the *postcoital*—after sex—*test* (PCT). Studies have demonstrated that this test is not a good predictor of sperm–mucus problems, though it is sometimes still used because it is easy and inexpensive. The couple are required to have intercourse at mid cycle and attend the clinic within 12–14 hours. A vaginal swab is taken and the interaction of the sperm and mucus is analysed in the lab. Most specialists these days prefer to use the Kremer test.

Hysterosalpingogram

A *Hysterosalpingogram* (HSG) is a way of looking at your fallopian tubes without undergoing surgery. The procedure is performed while you are awake. It is used to assess the health of your tubes—specifically, whether they are open and free of blockages or any obstructions that may prevent the smooth passage of your eggs. The openness of your tubes is referred to as *tubal patency.*

An HSG uses an x-ray to look at the uterus and internal outline of the fallopian tubes. It is usually done a few days after your last period when you are not ovulating and the lining of your uterus is thin. A speculum is inserted into the vagina through which a thin tube, a catheter, is passed into the cervix. A contrast medium or dye—a dense liquid that shows up on x-rays—is injected into the uterus. The flow of the dye can then be seen on a screen. The dye should flow through the fallopian tubes and out into the abdomen. By observing its course, the doctor can assess whether there are any significant blockages or obstructions in your tubes.

There are some problems with this procedure, however. Many women find it painful—enough to need some form of pain relief before and after—and the results may not be conclusive. In some instances, for example, the fallopian tube may have a muscle spasm, caused by the HSG itself, which temporarily blocks the course of the dye, so the tube appears to be blocked when it isn't. Sometimes there may appear to be a problem which, on further investigation, is found not to be the case, and vice versa. For these reasons some doctors now use sonohysterogram instead, and you may find this is used more commonly in the future.

Sonohysterogram

A sonohysterogram is a similar procedure that uses ultrasound rather than x-ray. It is also performed while you are awake. It can be done in the doctor's surgery or at a specialist ultrasound facility and it is generally less painful. A catheter is inserted via a speculum through the cervix and into the uterus, as with the HSG. Water or saline and dye is then inserted with gentle pressure, and its course through the fallopian tubes is monitored on a screen using ultrasound. Any obstruction or blockage can then be identified.

Laparoscopy

Your doctor may suggest performing a laparoscopy if the results of your clinical evaluation and the above tests are inconclusive. A laparoscopy is the most thorough and comprehensive way of examining your abdominal and pelvic cavities. It is also possible to treat some conditions at the time it is performed. Laparoscopy is a surgical procedure performed under general anaesthetic and therefore represents a step up in your level of treatment. It is something you should think about carefully and discuss in detail with your

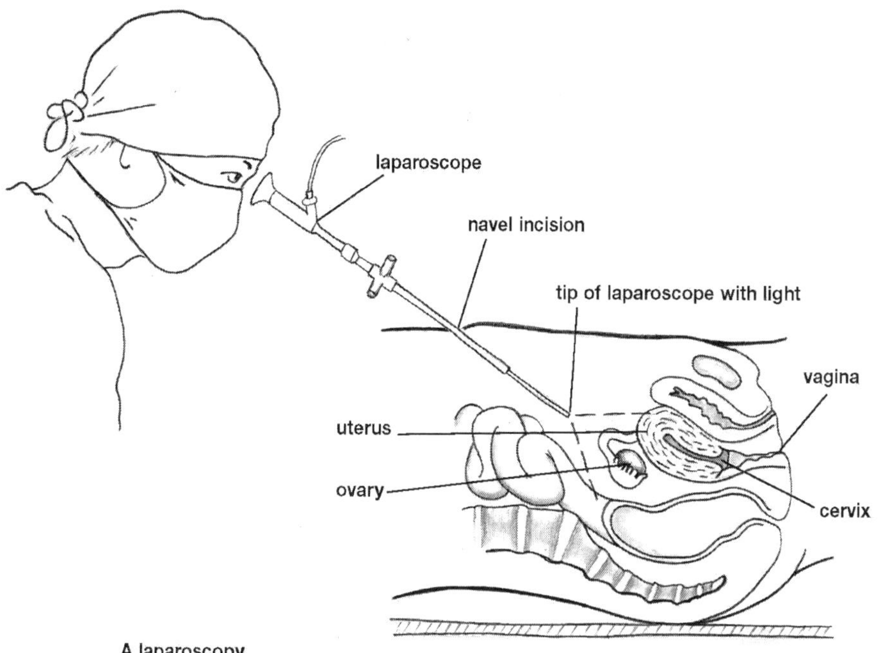

A laparoscopy

doctor before you proceed. It is a regularly performed, safe procedure, but, as with any surgery or procedure performed under a general anaesthetic, there are risks involved which your doctor should outline.

A laparoscopy is usually performed around mid-cycle, or when you have abstained from intercourse for a few days. This is to ensure there is no possibility of interfering with a pregnancy. The procedure is normally done at the day surgery of your clinic or local hospital. You will be told to fast from midnight the day before—or for about six hours prior to the procedure, depending on its scheduled time. Partners may drop you off, but are not normally expected to hang around. They will be given an estimated time to come and pick you up. You are not generally allowed to leave by yourself, and you are not allowed to drive. You may be able to get the phone number of the nurses' station so your partner can call to check when you are ready to be picked up. You are normally required to have four to five hours recovery time after the procedure. Occasionally, depending on your recovery, you may have to stay overnight.

As with any surgery, you will be asked to fill out a form giving details of your medical history and a nurse will run through a pre-surgery check. This includes checking your personal details, taking your blood pressure, temperature and weight. The nurse will ask you about allergies and medication, check the last time you had anything to eat or drink, and when you last went to the toilet. They will normally ask if you know exactly what is being done and whether you have any questions. You will be shown where to change and given a gown, hat and booties, and, if you haven't already, you must remove all your jewellery and make-up.

The anaesthetist will ask you some further questions regarding your medical and surgical history. They may ask whether you have had an anaesthetic before and whether you experienced any problems. They will ask you about anything relevant that you have noted on your medical history form. Your treating doctor may also check in with you and make sure you know exactly what is happening. You will be required to sign a form consenting to the surgery. When all this is done you will be wheeled into surgery.

THE PROCEDURE

The anaesthetist will insert a cannula—a small surgical tube—into your arm or the back of your hand through which the anaesthetic will be inserted. You may also have a light sedative or pre-med. While they are doing this, a nurse may stick some small patches on your chest. These enable the anaesthetist to monitor your vital signs—heart rate, blood pressure—throughout the surgery. Generally, there is a lot of discussion about the weather and the footy at this stage, to help you relax. Before you know it you are drifting off.

While you are sleeping soundly, a 1-centimetre incision is made in your belly button and a thin hollow needle, through which the doctor passes carbon dioxide gas, is inserted. The gas gently inflates the abdominal area, which allows the doctor to see your abdominal cavity more clearly. The needle is then withdrawn and the laparoscope is inserted through the same incision. The laparoscope is a kind of very fine telescope that is attached to a video camera, which enables the doctor to view your insides on a monitor. A further one or two small incisions may be made near your pubic hairline. The doctor will insert instruments through these incisions that will enable them to move your organs and ensure they can see everything clearly. They will then be able to do a thorough examination of your uterus, fallopian tubes and ovaries by watching the screen.

The doctor will pass a blue dye through your cervix, into your uterus and tubes—similar to the HSG and SonoHSG procedure. This will enable them to assess your tubal patency (the openness of your tubes). In addition, they will be able to see if you have any signs of:

- endometriosis
- ovarian cysts
- fibroids (non cancerous tumours made of fibrous tissue)
- scarring, adhesions or evidence of earlier infection
- congenital abnormalities
- polycystic ovaries.

If the doctor suspects there may be some abnormal tissue they may take a small sample of that tissue—a biopsy—for analysis in the lab.

The whole procedure normally takes approximately 15 to 20 minutes. When the doctor is done, you will be wheeled out of surgery and into recovery. You will wake feeling a little groggy, usually an hour or two later. It may take four to five hours for you to recover fully enough to go home. During this time the nurses will monitor your progress, check your level of pain or discomfort, provide medication where appropriate, and bring you a cup of tea and a sandwich or biscuit. You may experience any of the following after the procedure:

- a soreness around the site of your incisions, especially around your belly-button
- a feeling of swelling in the abdominal area, or pain similar to menstrual cramps
- a general feeling of being bloated—from the carbon dioxide gas—which may make it a little more difficult to breathe
- a referred pain in your shoulders or neck caused by the carbon dioxide gas
- nausea
- general muscular pain and tiredness
- some spotting or vaginal discharge, which may continue for a few days (you will need to use sanitary pads for this as you will be advised not to use tampons).

You will be advised to rest and take it easy for a few days afterwards. Most women will take some time off work—between one and three days is common, depending on your recovery and the sort of work you do. Once any discharge or bleeding has cleared up and the pain from your incisions wears off, you can go back to your usual physical and sexual activity, and to using tampons. Recovery rates vary, but it is completely normal not to feel 100 per cent for a week or so. Three or four days after surgery you will need to get your stitches removed—unless they are the sort that dissolve. Your local GP can do this. In some cases you may experience additional or persistent after-effects. If this is the case you should contact your doctor. These may include any of the following:

- increasing pain in the abdomen and vomiting
- persistent or bad smelling vaginal discharge
- heavy bleeding
- worse or persistent nausea
- pain when passing urine, or a feeling that you need to go often
- a fever or chills
- persistent pain, soreness or swelling around your incisions.

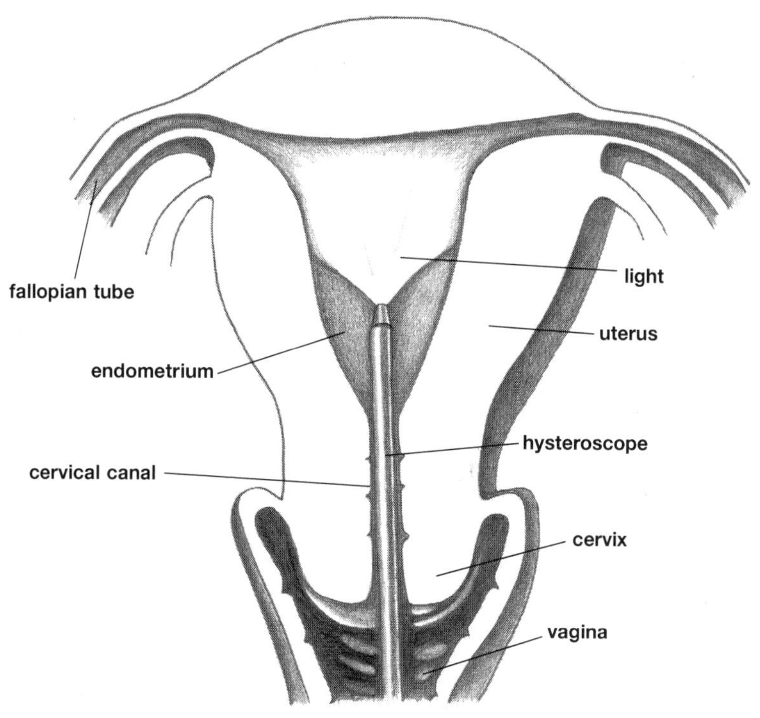

A hysteroscopy

Hysteroscopy

A hysteroscopy is an associated procedure which is usually performed under general anaesthetic at the same time as the laparoscopy. It can also be performed on its own in the doctor's surgery with a mild sedative rather than a general anaesthetic. It allows the doctor to examine the inside of your uterus using a similar telescope-like instrument—a hysteroscope—inserted directly into your uterus. This enables your doctor to see:

- the size, shape and position of your uterus
- the openings to your fallopian tubes

- any abnormal growths including fibroids or polyps (non-cancerous growths of the lining of the uterus)
- any evidence of cancer of the endometrium.

You will be asked to lie on your back with your legs open and supported—like a pap smear or scan. The doctor will place a speculum into your vagina and gently insert the hysteroscope into the uterus via the cervix. They may also insert some liquid or carbon dioxide gas which will enlarge the uterus and enable the doctor to see more clearly. As with the laparoscopy, the doctor may do a biopsy if they suspect you have some abnormal tissue. The whole procedure should take only a few minutes and you should be ready to go home after an hour or two. You can resume normal physical and sexual activity as soon as you feel well enough, and can use tampons as normal. You may experience some vaginal bleeding for a few days after the procedure, and some women experience period-type cramps.

Summing up

These early consultations will raise all sorts of issues for both partners, and it's important not to rush any decisions at this stage. Your doctor may give you some written material to take away, or may even have a video that explains your options. You will probably need to take some time to learn more about how reproduction works; most people know the basics, but not the details. This is a good time to start educating yourself.

You will also need to start dealing with how you feel about all this, and that means sitting down with your partner and talking opening and honestly. Your doctor may also suggest you see a clinic counsellor to discuss some of the issues that have arisen. It's not a requirement at this stage, but it is a good idea. The counsellors know a lot about infertility and how it affects people—probably much more than you do at this stage—and they can be a great resource and support.

The early stages of investigating infertility will look something like this:

- a pap smear and breast check with a GP or gynaecologist, Rubella and, in some cases, HIV and Hepatitis B and C tests
- a referral to an infertility specialist for a clinical evaluation, including a physical examination of both partners
- a blood test to check progesterone levels to assess ovulation
- a semen sample to analyse sperm
- a blood test to analyse levels of other significant hormones
- a kremer test to check sperm–mucus interaction
- a sonohysterogram or hysterosalpingogram to check internal reproductive health
- a laparoscopic investigation to determine tubal patency and identify other possible problems
- an initial chat with the clinic counsellor and/or a long chat with each other.

2 Preparing to make a baby

Health and lifestyle

For many couples, the first two or three visits to a specialist are a bit of a wake-up call—even just going to see an 'infertility specialist' makes everything more real all of a sudden. It's not just a lurking worry any more, but something you've actually got to address. It will take some time for your doctor to process the results of your tests and clinical evaluation, but this is not a bad thing. You will need this time to deal with some of the emotional consequences of starting down this path (see Chapter 9). Having a bit of time before you start any treatment also gives you the opportunity to start thinking about your general health and lifestyle.

If you do end up on some kind of treatment program there will be a whole range of lifestyle issues you'll have to address. This is not just because they may affect your capacity to conceive and carry a baby, but because they will affect your capacity to manage the program—especially in the long term. Being fit and healthy will certainly help you get through repeated treatment cycles. And, apart from anything else, it makes sense that if you're going to put a lot of energy and money into infertility treatment, you want to do everything you can to maximise your chances of conception and minimise the negative effects of treatment. You will want to feel you are doing everything possible to help. And, if you do conceive, you will want to be in the best possible shape.

There are a lot of things over which you have no control if you do start treatment, but the lifestyle factors are firmly in your hands: diet, exercise, smoking, drinking, caffeine intake, non-prescription drug use, work, leisure and stress. There is still a lot of misinformation about how each of these does and doesn't affect pregnancy, and it's important to be clear on the facts so you can make informed choices about your own behaviour. For some factors—smoking, for example—strong medical evidence tells us quite clearly it is not good for conception and not good for you or your unborn baby. For other factors—the effect of stress on conception—all sorts of claims are made, some based on little or no evidence. The information in this chapter aims to help you separate the myths from the facts. Once you've done that you can decide what, if any, changes you want to make to your lifestyle.

The key to all these lifestyle issues is balance; you don't have to turn yourself into some kind of super-fit health guru. Yes, it might be great if we all took up yoga and meditation, did regular exercise, replaced alcohol and caffeine with fresh juice and macrobiotic smoothies, ate bucket loads of organic fruit and veg and never touched another Mars Bar or Magnum, but we live in the real world. We lead busy lives with all sorts of demands and responsibilities that sometimes get in the way of our best intentions. There's no doubt that a good general level of health and fitness will help you through treatment—especially IVF—and it is really worth aiming for, but you have to decide what works for you and what you can successfully incorporate into your life. It's also worth remembering that whatever lifestyle changes you adopt, you may have to keep them up for three to six months, or three to six years. Your lifestyle needs to be healthy, but it also needs to be sustainable.

Having said that, whatever you decide, you need to give yourself permission to change your mind, to lapse, and to have a break or splurge between treatments. It's okay to have a glass of wine at night or a cappuccino at lunch. It's okay if your exercise plan goes down the tube. It's okay if you're flat out all week. The changes you make to your lifestyle are meant to help, not hinder; they're not supposed to become a burden.

Before I started treatment, I read that high levels of caffeine can negatively affect conception. So for my first five cycles I went completely caffeine free. I stopped drinking tea, coffee, Coke® and eating chocolate about a week before my egg pick-up and avoided them until after my pregnancy test result. I had a three-day headache every time. After twelve months or so, I was completely fed up with it. The caffeine withdrawal made me irritable and was just one more thing I had to worry about. I'd never really been a big coffee drinker anyway, and my caffeine levels were pretty low—probably low enough to not really have an effect on conception. I abandoned the plan, returned to my early morning cup of tea and occasional Flake, and felt much better for it. I know women who have given up caffeine for good because it makes them feel better. I know women for whom the thought of giving it up never crossed their minds. That's the thing, everyone approaches this in a different way; you need to check the facts and then decide what's best for you.

This chapter deals with the lifestyle factors that affect conception and pregnancy—smoking, alcohol consumption, caffeine intake, over-the-counter and prescription drugs, non-prescription drugs, diet, exercise, your weight and stress levels. It also includes the factors that may not directly affect conception, but have a significant impact on your capacity to manage your treatment, especially if you proceed to IVF—work and other responsibilities, leisure and relaxation, knowledge of infertility, financial considerations and privacy and support.

Smoking

Considerable scientific research demonstrates smoking has adverse effects on all stages of reproduction, including conception, growth and development in the uterus, miscarriage rates, birth and early childhood development. There is a direct link between the amount you smoke and the negative effects on you and your baby. If you are a heavy smoker you will do more damage than if you are a casual smoker, but all smoking does damage. Nicotine makes the blood vessels in your placenta constrict, which makes it more difficult for oxygen and essential nutrients to get through to your baby. Damage can occur to your baby at any stage during your pregnancy, but smoking in the second and third trimesters—three months and after—carries significant risks for your baby. Even if you don't smoke, but your partner does, you may experience passive smoking, which can also affect foetal development.

The effects of smoking, however, are reversible. If you stop smoking before you conceive, you avoid these negative consequences even if you have been smoking for many years. Your baby will benefit from your giving up smoking at any time during the pregnancy or after it is born. Scientific studies over past decades have shown that:

- in general, smokers suffer from infertility more than non-smokers and can take longer to conceive
- smoking can cause problems with your menstrual cycle that may affect your capacity to conceive
- problems with getting and maintaining an erection are more common in men who smoke
- smoking can reduce testosterone levels in men, which affects the development and quality of sperm

- smoking is associated with higher levels of miscarriage, spontaneous abortions and ectopic pregnancies
- smoking while you are pregnant is associated with premature births and low birth weights
- smoking during pregnancy increases the risk of complications at birth and Sudden Infant Death Syndrome (SIDS)
- heavy smokers have a higher chance of having babies with a cleft-palate or hare-lip.

If ever there was a good time to cut down or quit, this is it.

Many women find the nausea associated with the early stages of pregnancy helps them take the first step to quitting—drinking less coffee and alcohol can also help. As a start, the anti-smoking organisation *Quit* recommends 'The 4Ds: Drink water, Delay, Deep breathe, and Do something else'. It's always tough giving up, but there's plenty of help out there once you decide you want to.

Alcohol

Research suggests excessive or long-term alcohol use has significant adverse effects on conception and pregnancy, and frequent binge drinking, or getting drunk, can be harmful to you and your baby. Some studies have pointed to a link between alcohol consumption in women and the time taken to conceive, and some have suggested a link between alcohol consumption and higher rates of miscarriage. Excessive alcohol consumption in women can result in Foetal Alcohol Syndrome, a condition which can cause a range of congenital abnormalities in a baby.

However, the research does not suggest that the occasional glass of wine or beer will have any negative effect on you or your baby's health. Low levels of alcohol—a few standard drinks a week—are relatively safe. Having said that, many women decide to err on the side of caution anyway, and avoid alcohol completely during pregnancy.

In men, alcoholism is associated with impotence and decreased testosterone levels which can affect the number, development and motility of sperm. As with women, however, moderate alcohol is not believed to have any significant negative effect on fertility.

Caffeine

Some research studies have suggested a link between caffeine and gynaecological problems, miscarriage and birth defects. Some have suggested caffeine can cause a delay in conception, or that it can have a negative effect on the motility of sperm which reduces the sperm's capacity to reach and fertilise the egg. In all these studies, however, high levels of caffeine are believed to cause the problem; they are not caused by having an occasional coffee. However, caffeine is an artificial stimulant that can keep you awake, exacerbate anxiety and increase your blood pressure. Some women find that reducing the amount of caffeine in their diet makes them feel better, regardless of any effect it may have on their capacity to conceive and, as with alcohol, some err on the side of caution and give it up completely.

Coffee has the highest levels of caffeine—your cappuccino or latté has more than instant coffee. Caffeine is also found in tea—the longer you brew it the higher the level—and in hot chocolate and cocoa, Coke® and other cola-type drinks, and in chocolate. Most infertility specialists will advise you to keep an eye on your caffeine intake and ensure it stays within safe levels: no more than two cups of coffee or four cups of tea a day.

Drugs

You should discuss any drug use with your infertility specialist irrespective of whether the drug is an over-the-counter medication from the chemist, a prescription drug from your GP, or a non-prescription, street drug. In general, it is best to talk to your specialist before you take anything. You should definitely discuss any use of painkillers, antibiotics, anti-depressants, tranquillisers, sleeping pills, antacids, laxatives and vitamin supplements. It is especially important to let your doctor know if you are on medication for thyroid problems, diabetes, asthma, epilepsy or thrombosis.

There are a number of non-prescription, or 'street drugs'—marijuana, steroids, cocaine, heroin, methadone—that directly affect aspects of reproduction. Most also have a negative effect on your general health. It is not a good idea to be using any of these while you are trying to get pregnant, or undergoing treatment.

Marijuana

Marijuana is believed to have a direct negative affect on the menstrual cycle and ovulation. Studies show that regular users can have shorter cycles, especially shorter luteal phases (the second half of your cycle), which affects the chances of the fertilised egg implanting in the wall of the uterus. Long-term use of marijuana in men is associated with lower testosterone levels and a decrease in the quality and number of sperm.

Anabolic steroids

Anabolic steroids used to increase body and muscle mass can cause a range of general health problems. Regular use is associated with a reduced sperm function and a disruption of the normal workings of the male hormone system, both of which can result in decreased fertility.

Cocaine

Regular use of cocaine can impair the production of testosterone and sperm and can have a negative affect on the libido. Cocaine use in pregnancy is associated with low birth rates, bleeding from the placenta, premature birth and significant complications for newborns. Babies born to mothers who are regular cocaine users can suffer withdrawal.

Heroin and methadone

Narcotic-type drugs, including heroin and methadone, can have an indirect effect on ovulation by acting on the brain to inhibit dopamine (a hormone secreted by the brain) and causing an increase in prolactin. Regular heroin use is also likely to be associated with poor nutrition, weight loss and increased risk of infectious diseases as well as poor general health, all of which will have a negative effect on the capacity to conceive.

Naturopaths and alternative health practitioners

There is a broad range of alternative health practitioners who can provide advice on diet, exercise, stress management and general and reproductive health. Some women find them enormously helpful, some prefer to just stick with their medical specialist. If you do consult an alternative practitioner while you are undergoing other treatment, make sure you tell your infertility specialist about them, and tell your alternative practitioner about your infertility specialist. If everyone knows what's happening, there is less chance of a problem arising. If you are taking any kind of Chinese, herbal, naturopathic or homeopathic remedy—however benign you think it might be—you should tell your infertility specialist.

Diet

A good, balanced diet will make you feel better, give you more energy and enable you to recover from surgical procedures more quickly. It will help your immune system work more effectively, and will help keep illness and infection at bay. The benefits of a healthy diet will be felt during pregnancy and passed on to your baby. This might be a good time to look at what you eat and make some adjustments if necessary.

A broad rule of thumb for a healthy diet is to have a moderate intake of complex carbohydrate and protein and a low intake of fat and sugar. Your diet should be rich in fibre with adequate vitamins and minerals. This means lots of fresh fruit and vegetables, cereals, rice, noodles, pasta, beans, lentils and bread, and regular servings of fish, poultry, tofu or soy products. It means fewer pies, pizzas, battered fish and chips, take-away burgers and fried food, and less butter, cream, cakes and sweets. You should also drink plenty of water every day. Everyone differs, of course, and you may want to do some further research, or consult a dietician or naturopath to give you more personalised advice. There are many good books that deal with diet and conception and pregnancy.

Some women take a pre-conception or pregnancy vitamin supplement. Dieticians generally suggest it is better to get your vitamins and minerals directly from food, but if your diet is not particularly good, or you have some specific dietary restrictions, a supplement may be a sensible solution. However, there is no evidence that vitamin supplementation is necessary for optimum fertility. The exception to this is folic acid (see below).

There are some specific dietary considerations relating to conception and pregnancy, including consumption of foods containing folic acid, B vitamins, vitamins A, C and E (anitoxidants), calcium, iron and fatty acids.

Folic acid

Folic acid is probably the most important single addition you can make to your diet. If you do nothing else, buy a folic acid supplement and start taking it straightaway. Check with your doctor or the pharmacist about the correct dosage. Folic acid has been shown to significantly lower the risk of neural tube defects in babies, especially spina bifida. Good sources of folic acid are wholegrain cereals, lentils, chickpeas, kidney beans and spinach. However, in this case, taking a supplement is recommended.

B vitamins

Vitamins B6 and B12 are important for the overall health of women generally, and particularly pregnant women and women trying to conceive. They are necessary for metabolising protein and carbohydrates. Good sources of B6 are meat, liver and grains. Good sources of B12 are fish, eggs, meat and milk. If you are a vegetarian you may need to pay particular attention to your B12 intake.

Vitamins A, C and E

These vitamins are antioxidants, which are important for strengthening your immune system and protecting your body against infection and disease. Vitamin C also helps the body to absorb iron. Some studies have shown a link between antioxidants and fertility; for example, a deficiency of vitamin E may result in a decrease in sperm motility, and low levels of vitamin C may result in fewer, slower or abnormally shaped sperm. Some studies have suggested vitamin C is important in making sure the ovaries function correctly, though this does necessarily mean an increased intake will be beneficial.

Good sources of vitamin A are meat, eggs, liver and butter, and good sources of beta-carotene—the water-soluble form of vitamin A—are carrots, apricots, pumpkin and spinach. Some studies have suggested a link between too much vitamin A and cleft palate. It is probably best to avoid vitamin A supplements. Most pregnancy multi-vitamins do not include vitamin A. Vitamin C is found in useful amounts in a variety of fruits and vegetables, including, oranges, tomatoes, strawberries, broccoli, sweet potato and capsicum. Vitamin E is found primarily in seed oils, such as corn oil or safflower oil, and in almonds, hazelnuts, sunflower seeds, peanut butter and salmon. It is difficult to get large quantities of vitamin E from food, and if you do need to increase your vitamin E intake, you might have to take a supplement. Discuss it with your doctor first.

Calcium

Calcium helps to maintain strong bones and good muscle function and it's important you go into any pregnancy with healthy levels of calcium in your body. Once you are pregnant, your baby will draw on your calcium store to build its skeleton, and you will also need it to make sure your bones remain strong. Good sources of calcium are milk, cheese, cottage cheese and yoghurt (but see the section on 'Listeria' on p. 45). Calcium is also found in lesser amounts in leafy vegetables, wholegrains, nuts and pulses.

Iron

Iron is essential for the production of haemoglobin, which transports oxygen to the placenta. During pregnancy your baby will draw on your reserves of iron, which is why it is important to maintain good iron levels while you are trying to conceive. If your iron levels are low and you are anaemic you may need to take an iron supplement before or during your infertility treatment. Check with your doctor. Good sources of iron are lean red meat, green leafy vegetables, raisins, prunes, dried apricots, nuts and lentils.

Fatty acids

Fatty acids ensure the development and functioning of body tissues including kidney, liver, heart, blood vessels and brain. A deficiency in fatty acids has been associated with reduced fertility. It is particularly important to have a good intake of Omega-3 fatty acids, which influence a range of important body functions. Good sources of Omega-3s are oily fish, including tuna, salmon, pilchards, sardines and trout, and also linseed, canola or soya bean oil and pumpkin seeds.

Listeria and other bacteria

Listeria is a bacteria found in certain foods. It has sometimes been associated with pregnancy loss. It is relatively uncommon, however, especially in women who are healthy, have a good diet and access to quality fresh and refrigerated foods. To be safe, once you have had a positive pregnancy test, you should avoid eating any soft and blue-veined cheeses, including brie, camembert and ricotta—though these are all okay if cooked and served hot. You should also steer clear of rare or cured meats, paté, uncooked eggs (including mayonnaise and Caesar salads), barbecued chickens, serve-yourself salads, cold meats from the deli counter and any reheated food. You should avoid contact with raw meat and be thorough about washing chopping boards and utensils. As a precaution, you should make sure you wash all fruit and vegetables thoroughly too.

Exercise

The fitter and stronger you are when you begin treatment, the more able your body will be to cope with the various drugs and procedures; you will feel less knocked about generally and will recover more quickly. Regular, moderate exercise helps you sleep, strengthens your bones, reduces body fat, increases your endorphins and helps to protect you against a broad range of illnesses.

As there is always some lead-in time to treatment, now is a good time to start thinking about the exercise you do, or don't do. Again, there's no need to take up kick-boxing or start long-distance running, but 20 minutes a day—or every other day—will make a difference. Walking, cycling and swimming are good—cheap, easy and fun—team sports or low-impact aerobics are also good; as is any kind of yoga, or stretching or strengthening exercise.

You may find that your infertility treatment has an impact on the sort of exercise you do and how often you do it. I used to always run, not excessively, but a gentle 20-minute jog a few days a week. Once I started the injections I stopped. Certainly, there was a physical reaction to the hormones—I was more tired and started to experience some abdominal discomfort—but it was more an emotional response; it just didn't seem a good idea to bounce my dozen or so developing follicles around the park. I walked instead, and found that much more comfortable and quite relaxing. In between cycles I used to go back to running, but after a while, after repeated cycles, I found I just didn't have the energy. The walking stayed with me though.

It is generally advisable to avoid any exercise that causes a prolonged rise in your body temperature or significant increase in your pulse rate. Working up a slight sweat is fine, but intensive aerobic exercise that increases your heart rate, makes you go red, or causes you to sweat profusely should be avoided. Although the evidence in relation to pregnancy is inconclusive, it is generally sensible to keep your pulse below 140. This is especially important during the waiting period after an embryo transfer, when you do not yet know whether you are pregnant.

There is a connection between exercise and infertility, but only where that exercise is excessive. Marathon runners, gymnasts, dancers, elite athletes and people who do daily high-level aerobic exercise to maintain a particular body weight or shape may experience problems. Excessive exercise in women can upset the natural hormone balance and can cause disruptions to your cycle, which affects your ovulation and hence your capacity to conceive. Over-exercising is associated with irregular periods and the absence of periods. If you are not in these categories (marathon runner, elite athlete, etc.)—even if you consider yourself to be quite 'sporty'—you are unlikely to experience these problems.

Men who exercise excessively may produce less testosterone or suffer from over-heated testes, which can affect the production of sperm. Again though, for most men enjoying normal sporting activities—a game of squash a couple of times a week, working out at the gym, or a game of footy on the weekend—there's nothing to worry about.

Weight

For most women within a broad normal range, weight will not be a factor in conception. Maintaining a consistent, healthy weight and avoiding significant fluctuations in your weight is important—this is not a time to be exploring new or fad diets. However, there is a connection between being significantly over- or underweight and infertility. If you are underweight you are more at risk of menstrual dysfunction—having irregular periods, or no periods at all. If your body fat is very low (less than 10 per cent) your ovaries may not function normally and your ovulation will be affected. There is a high correlation between eating disorders—anorexia nervosa and bulimia—and problems with fertility.

Being overweight can also cause disruptions to the menstrual cycle because of an imbalance of hormones, and is associated with the development of insulin resistance in women with polycystic ovarian syndrome (PCOS) (see Chapter 3), which can affect ovulation. Being overweight makes ovarian stimulation difficult, and some aspects of treatment—egg retrieval and embryo transfer, for example—are more difficult to perform in severely overweight women.

Stress

Stress can be a factor in conception, but not in the way many people believe. Most women who are struggling with their fertility or undergoing some kind of treatment have been told at one time or another to 'relax'—after all *if you just stop worrying, you'll get pregnant* (probably the *No.1 Most Irritating Comment*). Though many people believe it, and often say it, there is just no medical evidence to suggest that worrying about getting pregnant will in any way stop you getting pregnant, or that not worrying about it will help you get pregnant. Certainly, there is medical evidence to suggest links between a person's emotional and physical wellbeing, but not enough is known in the case of infertility to draw broad conclusions. There *is* a relationship between stress and conception, but it is very specific.

Research suggests that significant psychological stress in a woman can affect ovulation. Where the stress is extreme, a woman can suffer anovulation (no ovulation) or amenorrhea (the absence of periods). If the stress occurs around mid-cycle there may be a negative effect on that cycle's ovulation. For stress to affect ovulation, however, it needs to be extreme (war, trauma for example; ordinary, everyday worries do not cause this. If you feel stressed from work or family, or even from the treatment, but are ovulating normally, you really don't need to worry.

Significant stress in men can cause a lower sperm count because stress hormones can have a negative effect on the production of testosterone, which is necessary for the formation of sperm. Again, though, this is not everyday stress about work or family, but extreme stress.

Probably the most common and significant way in which stress influences conception is in the frequency of sex. A busy, highly stressed couple is likely to have less sex than a couple who is relaxed and has more leisure time. Perhaps if you do have a relaxing, romantic dinner—followed by sex—or a week's holiday by the beach—incorporating lots of sex—you might get pregnant, but this is not because of some mysterious magical mind–body connection, but because you spent more time in bed together.

The adoption myth

We have all heard the story of the friend of a friend who was trying to conceive for years and then adopted a child, and hey! six months later she was pregnant naturally! In fact, there have been a number of studies—comparing similar couples who have adopted and not adopted—that clearly demonstrate the chances of conception are higher among those couples who do *not* adopt. Adopting couples—with a baby or child to look after, and less urgency to conceive—generally have less sex, while the non-adopting couples continue to have more frequent sex. Unless there is a major impediment to conception in these couples, more sex means a greater chance of having a baby.

Lifestyle and managing treatment

Starting treatment can be an anxious time, but most people go into it with a reasonable degree of optimism and energy. A simple course of drugs, or a relatively minor surgical procedure may be all you need—or you may be looking at a cycle of IVF treatment. If you conceive on your first or second cycle, the impact of the treatment will probably be less than if you undergo four, five or more cycles. However long you're having treatment, it's a big commitment and you will most likely have to make a few adjustments to your lifestyle. The key to this is finding the right balance between giving the treatment priority, and not letting it take over your life. This is where it's really important to look at all the other factors that make up your life: work, family, leisure and money.

Work and other responsibilities

There is no reason why a couple can't incorporate infertility treatment into their two full-time careers. But if you do IVF, it will take a bit of organisation and planning, and you can expect a few teething problems at first while you become familiar with the routines. Most clinics are used to the fact that these days both partners work. For this reason, they normally have surgeries early in the morning so you can have injections, blood tests or see your doctor before work. Inevitably, though, there will be occasions when you need to take time off—either for a procedure, or maybe for a mental health day after a cancelled cycle, a negative result, or a miscarriage.

You will need to give some thought to who, if anyone, you tell at work and when you tell them. In the early stages at least, you can probably keep your treatment private through a combination of out-of-hours' appointments and sick leave. Most clinics recognise the importance of discretion, and will provide medical certificates that are deliberately non-specific. Difficulties might arise though if, for example, you need to leave suddenly in the middle of the day for an injection, or if you take longer than expected to recover from a surgical procedure.

One of the biggest difficulties is the fact that, whatever your treatment, it is governed by your menstrual cycle. Hormone stimulation can be quite variable and it's almost impossible to be specific about when you will need time off. Things also become more difficult the longer you are involved in treatment, especially as your sick leave entitlements get used up, or your occasional late starts and disappearances begin to be noticed. Many women use their annual leave for treatment, especially those who have to travel long distances to a clinic or stay overnight.

The biggest mistake I made was not telling the people I worked with. I hid it as if it was a failure. It was a mistake because the staff working for me really didn't understand why some days I just wasn't concerned about the small things in life. I should have been absolutely open. I can say that now. And I would be now. It wasn't until I met someone who was very open about the whole thing that I realised it doesn't have to be a secret. How she dealt with it—with people knowing—was a lot better. So I think that was one of my biggest mistakes, keeping it to myself.

I realised how lonely I was when I was doing the treatment. My husband was there for me and we did talk about it a lot, but I didn't know any other women who were going through it, so I didn't have anyone else to talk to. I wasn't interested in going to 'IVF Friends' or anything like that. I just wanted someone who I could go to lunch with and say, 'This is crap I'm shoving up my nose,' and she'd say, 'Yeah it is. I know what you mean.'

Tanya

How you handle all of this will, of course, depend on your type of job and your relationship with your employer. Most men will probably not want to discuss the latest round of treatment with their work mates over lunch and, because they do not generally have the treatment, will not need to take so much time off. But, they may need to accompany you to an appointment, or pick you up after a procedure. Women, on the other hand, may want to talk about it more, and will certainly have to take time off. If your boss knows what's happening and is supportive it can be a real help; you don't have to make up excuses if your energy levels fluctuate or have to explain changes in your moods or routines. Most of all, it can take the strain out of planning ahead when you're not really sure what days you are going to need to take off. One way to handle it might be to make a general statement—to one or two people—about the fact that you are having infertility treatment at the start, and then share whatever details you are comfortable with later on.

Work can play a very positive role in managing your treatment, and some women throw themselves into it as a way of diverting attention from their infertility. It can be a distraction on days when you are waiting for test results or are anxious about your next procedure. It can be a consistent and reliable influence in your life when not much else is. It can provide an easy social environment where you forget about hormone levels and temperature charts for a while and talk about the latest office drama. It can provide positive affirmation at a time when your self-esteem might be taking a battering.

There can be negatives, too—if your job is very stressful, if you really don't enjoy it, or if you work long hours—these will make managing your treatment more difficult. If there are things you can do to improve your working day, cut down your hours, or alleviate the stress, they're worth doing before starting treatment. This may not be a good time to take on a promotion or any new or additional responsibilities. In fact, if possible, it's a good time to off-load, to delegate, to practise saying 'No'. If things are really tough you might think about going part-time to give yourself a little more flexibility and the opportunity to rest and recover after each cycle. This has to be balanced, of course, by your financial situation and the fact that, with treatment, you are facing a number of additional expenses.

Most of us have other responsibilities outside work—family, social clubs, sports teams, political affiliations, volunteer work, evening classes or part-time study. Again, these can be a positive or a negative. If they are good for you, fun and a distraction, hang onto them; if they tire you out, frustrate you or are a burden, try to wind them down or off-load them. If possible, avoid any major changes or disruptions to your life while you're undergoing treatment, especially at the beginning when it's all quite new. It's not a good time, for example, to move house, do major renovations, start a course, retrain, expand your business, or anything else that diverts significant energy from dealing with the effects of infertility and its treatment.

> I pretty much told all the girls I worked with, mostly because it was impossible to go through treatment without people knowing. A few people said to me, 'You don't have to tell work everything,' but I thought 'No, I'm going to tell everyone,' and I was really glad I did.
>
> Hannah

Leisure and relaxation

Infertility treatment—especially IVF—demands a slower pace and a bit more down-time. It is not really compatible with a very active social life. A combination of the emotional demands and the physical effects of the drugs will leave you with less energy. This doesn't mean you have to turn into a hermit and never go out, but how often you go out, and the sort of things you enjoy doing might change. Many couples find they experience a subtle shift in their social life to lower-energy, quieter or more home-based activities. You might not feel like hosting a big dinner or barbecue, or have the energy to haul yourself across town to a party. Depending on the sort of treatment you are having, you may require injections at a specific time which will limit what you can do. You wouldn't be the first couple to sneak away from your host's dining table to draw up hormone injections in their bathroom, but alternatively, you might just choose to stay at home on those days.

The people you socialise with might also shift a little. Friends who are pregnant, have babies or small children, or with whom you just don't feel particularly comfortable around this subject, might take a back seat for a while. As you start treatment you may well find other infertility patients pop up where you least expect—a woman on your hockey team, someone who works down the corridor, an old school friend. Some days, a lunch or dinner with people who are going through the same things as you is just that much easier.

> For me it was a good thing telling people. It was something I had to get off my chest. If I hadn't it would have been worse when people said insensitive things like, 'Oh so when are you two going to have a baby'. At least, when they knew . . . they still said things that would piss me off, but at least if I ever snapped people would cut me more slack. The other issue is that some of the protocols actually interfere with when you can be at a particular place and its disrespectful to your friends to say, 'Oh, we can't be there until such and such a time', and not give a reason. If they know you're on IVF, they know you're having injections or whatever, it makes it easier. If people know, if it's an open conversation, you know what's going on, they know what's going on, its better for all concerned. Also, I told a friend who then told me of someone else who was going on IVF and that way I was able to make a new friendship with someone going through the same thing at the same time. If I had never said anything, that would never have happened.
>
> Andrea

Making the most of your leisure time—and spending part of that time with your partner—is an important part of managing treatment. It's easy to get bogged down by the constant round of drugs, tests and procedures, and you need to build in regular fun and relaxing activities with your partner, friends and family— picnics in the park, trips to the beach, a visit to the movies or footy are essential distractions.

Privacy and support

For most couples, doubts about their fertility are not something they want to discuss openly, especially at first. It's enough to have to talk about all sorts of private and intimate things with the doctor or nurses. It is certainly possible to keep your treatment private, and many couples choose to do this. However, if you do end up doing

IVF, you will be having daily injections, taking regular trips to a clinic, and occasional visits to a hospital or day-surgery, so it may be difficult to maintain complete privacy from people with whom you have very regular contact.

Many couples decide not to tell friends or other family members for a variety of reasons. Infertility is, in large part, about sex, which for most people is a private matter not usually discussed outside the partnership. A diagnosis of infertility may be accompanied by a range of emotions: shame, embarrassment, anxiety, guilt, anger or frustration, which many couples feel are best dealt with between themselves, or with a counsellor. Some people find that others knowing can be a burden and that well-meant questions about how your treatment is progressing, or whether you've had the results of a test, just add to the pressure you feel. You might find that lots of people are poorly informed about infertility and its treatment, therefore they say or do things that really aren't helpful—you can do without inappropriate or upsetting comments, and you won't generally have the energy or patience to educate them.

The flip side of all this is that it might actually be good if a few people know what is happening, perhaps your mum, sister, best friend, close colleague or neighbour. Having other people to talk to is really important, and can take the pressure off you and your partner. Apart from anything else, there's a steep learning curve involved in infertility treatment and it can be helpful to have someone to read the leaflets and books with you. There may be occasions when your partner can't make it to the hospital on time and you need to have someone to pick you up and keep an eye on you during the afternoon while you recover from the anaesthetic. Sometimes you might just need to talk through how you feel, have a hug, or cry on someone's shoulder. Men and women will probably deal with this issue differently; men may prefer just to discuss it with their partners, or share it with a brother or close friend.

The majority of people I spoke to or interviewed while writing this book came down on the side of telling at least a few people,

> I called a friend back home and as soon as I mentioned I had a low sperm count she just kind of said, 'Oh yeah', and then totally changed the subject and has never mentioned it since. Then I told another friend who did the exact same thing. She said, 'Oh you've just got married, enjoy the time while you have it, just the two of you.' Then I called another friend of mine, he and his wife were having some problems as well, so we actually had a bit of a chat. Then they actually got pregnant and he has never mentioned it since. After that we got the impression that some people just don't want to know.
>
> We got some information about IVF from the counsellors to give to our families to read, basically about what we had been going through. In one of them it says, 'Things not to say to the couple'. You know, 'to go on holiday', 'to have a nice dinner with a glass of wine', 'to relax'. When we told my sister she said a few times, 'You have to believe in the power of positive thinking', things like that. And people always have these stories about couples who have been through IVF for eight years and had no luck and then they get pregnant . . . and I'm like . . . I just sit there smiling going, 'Yeah, yeah', and thinking, 'You have no idea'.
>
> Charles

especially at work. They felt that having a support network was essential, and where that support was shared between family and friends or colleagues, it was even better. On balance, for them, the benefits of other people knowing far outweighed any negatives. Like everything else, though, it's a matter of weighing up the various pros and cons and deciding for yourselves.

Money

Some infertility treatment—especially IVF—is expensive and, depending on your income, these expenses will be more or less of a

> Talking to other people who had gone through it, that was such a support and so informative because, no matter what you read or what the nurses tell you, it's great to have other people who've done it. It's so different to what you read in the clinic manual because they can't really cover everything in detail. It says, 'Day 1 you do this, and day 2 you do that', but what's involved in that one thing—whether it's the emotional or physical—is just so much. In your head it's like, 'Oh yes, that's a procedure, I can understand that', but it's different when you are actually doing it. It was very much more complicated than it appeared.
>
> Tracy

burden—almost everyone feels the impact in one way or another. Many people take time off between IVF cycles, not just to allow their bodies to recover, but also to save up for the next one. Some people manage five or six cycles in a year, especially if some of those are thaw cycles and therefore less expensive. Some people might only be able to afford to do one. If your treatment extends over a number of years, you might find yourselves using your savings, borrowing money, or prioritising treatment over your annual holiday or other things. It is likely your ordinary, everyday spending will be a bit tight, your social activities curtailed, decorating the house will be put on hold, and the trip interstate or overseas will fall by the wayside.

Irrespective of your particular financial circumstances, money can be a source of stress between the two of you, and may become more so if you do repeated cycles without success. Inevitably, you start to total up the cost of treatment and think about all the other things you could do with the money. As with everything else, it's important to keep the channels of communication open and make sure you discuss problems with your partner as and when they arise.

Learning about infertility

Most people have a basic understanding of how everything works, but in order to understand the various tests and diagnoses, and to make informed choices about your treatment, you need to know more than that. The more complex your treatment, the more you need to know. You need to understand how ovulation works, what sperm does exactly and how it all comes together to produce an embryo that implants. You need to know a bit about anatomy—fallopian tubes, ovaries and testes—and the alphabet soup of hormones, FSH, LH, HCG, and more.

A good basic knowledge will make you feel more confident when you are with your specialist, and will enable you to know what questions to ask and to understand the answers. You will feel more empowered, more able to explore different options and more on top of your treatment generally. The next few chapters of this book will help, but there are other sources. Read everything your specialist gives you, rifle the racks of brochures at the clinic, go to your local library, look up 'reproduction' in an encyclopaedia, check the clinic websites, talk to other people with infertility problems and share the information with each other.

Summing up

Infertility is a complex business and many people are completely overwhelmed when they first come up against it.

A good preparation for infertility treatment, especially IVF, will include:

- talking through how you feel about starting treatment and exploring the issues it raises for you, as individuals and as a couple
- acknowledging there are going to be some emotional and physical demands made on you both requiring some adjustments to your lifestyle

- doing some regular exercise, eating well and drinking less alcohol and caffeinated drinks
- giving up smoking
- starting a course of folic acid
- scaling down work or other responsibilities and building some down-time into your lives
- reading around the subject of reproduction and infertility and talking to other people
- thinking about who you are going to tell and who's going to be in your support network
- doing some careful budgeting and saving money
- keeping open the channels of communication with your partner and discussing issues as they comes up.

The more of these things you can incorporate into your lives, the better able you will be to manage your infertility and its treatment.

> If I'd had a good support network from the start, that would have helped. A group of people going through the same thing makes a huge difference. Also, the clinic offers free counselling and I never took it up because I've always been very dismissive of that sort of thing—we both are—but I possibly should have taken advantage of that.
>
> Andrea

3

Causes of infertility

Finding some answers

Finding out why you've been having problems conceiving can be a bit scary, but it can also be an enormous relief. The most important thing to bear in mind at this early stage is that treatment is available for a wide range of problems. These days, it is highly unlikely you will hear the dreaded, 'I'm sorry, you can't have children'. For women of our mother's generation, certain conditions—blocked fallopian tubes being the most common—meant an end to their hopes of bearing children. In vitro fertilisation changed that.

Advances in infertility treatment—including IVF—over the past two decades and, more recently, developments in the treatment of male infertility, mean that few conditions result in absolute sterility. Even in the worst instances—where there are no eggs or no sperm—it may be possible to conceive using the eggs or sperm of a donor. It is far more likely, though, you will have a problem with ovulation, with hormone levels, blocked tubes, or a problem with the quality or quantity of sperm—all of which may be treatable.

Is it also quite possible your specialist won't uncover any specific cause as to why you aren't conceiving. In some ways this, too, can be a relief—there's nothing actually wrong with either of you and maybe you just need to give it more time—but it can also be quite frustrating, especially if you've been trying for a while. Sometimes the problem might be a combination of quite subtle factors rather than one specific thing. Just because your doctor can't pinpoint the exact problem, though, doesn't mean they can't help. You may still benefit from treatment.

Irrespective of your diagnosis—or lack of it—finding out the results of all the tests and investigations can be an anxious time. It certainly helps if you have some idea of what to expect and you understand that a low sperm count or irregular periods is not the end of the story. It might just be that achieving a successful pregnancy is going to be a little more complicated than you imagined.

Causes of infertility in women include problems with hormones and ovulation, problems relating to the fallopian tubes and uterus, problems arising as a result of age and, less commonly, problems with sex. Also, some women can conceive easily enough but, for a variety of reasons, are unable to carry a baby to term (see Chapter 5). Causes of infertility in men include problems with hormones and sperm, problems relating to the penis or testes, the reproductive glands and ducts and, again less commonly, problems with sex. There is also a specific diagnosis—relating to the couple—called *idiopathic* infertility, where none of these apply and the cause is unknown.

In order to understand the causes of infertility—when things go wrong—you need to understand what happens when everything goes right. The biology of how it all happens is actually quite complex, and it's worth taking a bit of time to try and get your heads around it. If you can get a basic grasp of the process it will really help later if you end up having more complex treatment.

How a baby is made

The successful coming together of an egg and sperm to produce an embryo that implants in the uterus and later develops into a baby is governed by the actions of a number of different hormones. Hormones are chemical messengers that flow through the blood stream from one part of the body to another. These hormones are controlled by the hypothalamus, a part of the brain located roughly behind the nose.

Let's begin with the woman.

The hypothalamus produces gonadotrophin-releasing hormone (GnRH), which it sends to the pituitary gland situated just beneath it. The GnRH lets the pituitary gland know it is time to release follicle stimulating hormone (FSH) and luteinising hormone (LH), two key hormones that control the development and release of the eggs, and the production of oestrogen and progesterone. The main oestrogen naturally produced by the body is called *oestradiol*. The pituitary gland also produces prolactin, which is responsible for stimulating milk production after pregnancy.

All pre-menopausal women have a supply of eggs that they were born with stored in their ovaries. These eggs are in a kind of sac, called a follicle, that protects and supports them. Each month, when the hypothalamus sends its message to the pituitary gland to start producing FSH, the FSH prompts the ovaries to start developing some of these follicles. At the same time as the follicles and the eggs inside them are growing, the ovaries are starting to produce oestrogen, the key female hormone responsible for stimulating growth.

As the oestrogen level rises, the pituitary gland starts to secrete less FSH, just enough, in fact, to support one 'dominant' follicle to develop further. The oestrogen, meanwhile, is causing the lining of the uterus (the *endometrium*) to thicken in preparation for receiving a fertilised egg. When the oestrogen rises to a certain level the pituitary gland releases the luteinising hormone, which in turn signals the ovaries to start ovulating—that is, to release its egg. This is known as the *LH surge* and it can be detected by testing the woman's

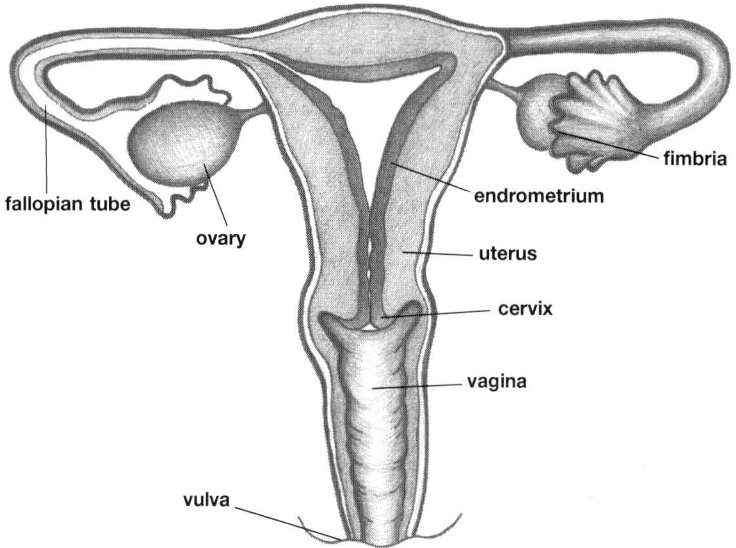

The female reproductive system

blood or urine. Ovulation will occur 24 to 36 hours after the LH surge. This is the time you need to have sex—or do an insemination—if you are aiming to conceive. Just before this ovulation occurs mucus forms in the cervix providing a nurturing environment in which to receive the sperm. This whole process takes about two weeks and is called the *proliferative* or *follicular phase* of the menstrual cycle.

At ovulation, the egg is released from the follicle and picked up by the *fimbria*—little tentacles at the opening of the fallopian tube. The ovaries continue to produce oestrogen, but in smaller quantities. After ovulation the empty follicle that contained the egg—now called the *corpus luteum*—starts to produce progesterone, the other key female reproductive hormone. Progesterone causes the endometrium—the lining of the uterus—to stop thickening and

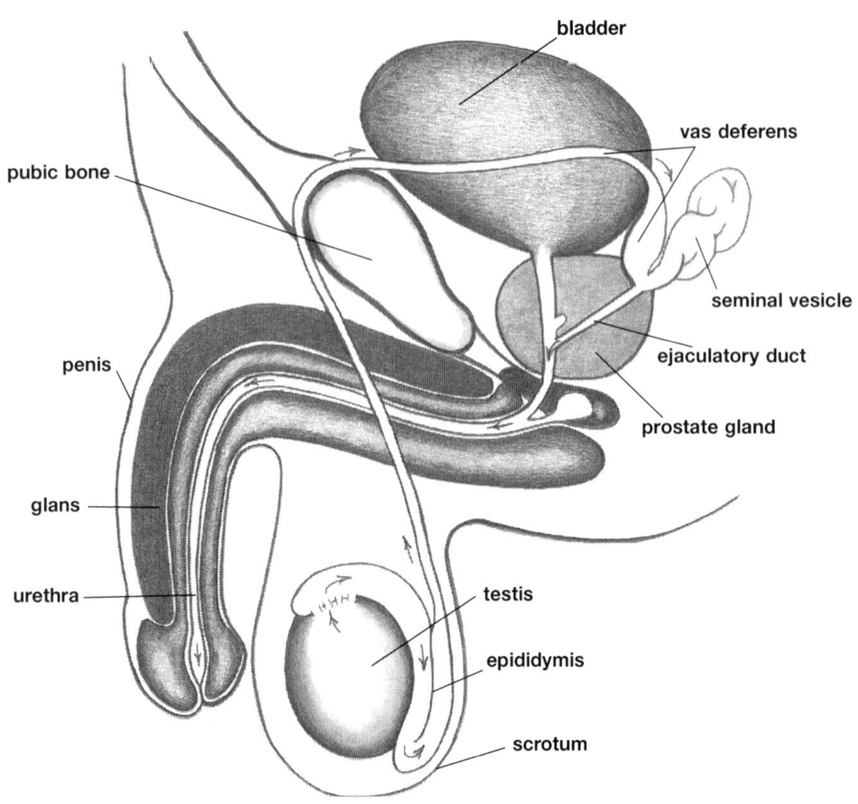

The male reproductive system

become receptive to an embryo. At this point the unfertilised egg is floating around the fallopian tube waiting to meet up with a sperm.

Meanwhile, the man is preparing to play his part. Unlike women who are born with their eggs, men manufacture sperm on an ongoing basis. The pituitary gland sends out FSH which, in men, stimulates the production of sperm in the testes, and LH which stimulates the production of testosterone. Testosterone is the key male reproductive hormone and it has a range of functions, including helping with the healthy production of sperm. As the sperm mature, they move from the testes to the *epididymis*, a small organ, where they develop their movement or motility. In the epididymis the tails of the sperm mature and the sperm take on their characteristic tadpole shape. It is the rapid movement of the tail that will later enable the sperm to swim towards the egg.

The sperm then move from the epididymis to the *vas deferens*, a thin tube that leads to the *seminal vesicles*, and the *ejaculatory duct*, which is adjacent to the prostate gland. The seminal vesicle is where the fluid that makes up most of the ejaculate is produced. The mature sperm stay in the vas deferens until the man ejaculates. When this happens, the sperm mixes with the fluid from the seminal vesicles creating semen. The semen—containing millions of sperm—is expelled through the *urethra*, and passed into the woman's vagina during ejaculation.

The sperm then begin to make their way through the cervix of the woman, into the uterus and up towards the fallopian tube where the egg is waiting. Many of the sperm will die along the way, with only a few hundred actually making it to the fallopian tube. Sperm can survive for at least one to two days inside the woman but the egg is only able to be fertilised for approximately 12 to 24 hours. This is a woman's fertile time—the window of opportunity.

The egg meets the sperm and the head of the sperm penetrates the egg's hard outer shell—the *zona pellucida*—and fertilises the egg. The tail of the sperm drops off and the fertilised egg makes its way to the uterus where it implants into the prepared endometrium. It takes approximately five days for the fertilised *embryo* to reach and implant into the endometrium. If the implantation is successful, human chorionic gonadotrophin (HCG), the pregnancy hormone, is produced. It is HCG in a blood or urine test that confirms you are pregnant.

If the egg fails to fertilise, or the embryo fails to implant in the endometrium, it passes through the uterus and out of the body, or it may be reabsorbed in the menstrual fluid. The *endometrium* is then shed as menstruation (the period). Once the progesterone levels have dropped, the hypothalamus then sends GnRH to the pituitary

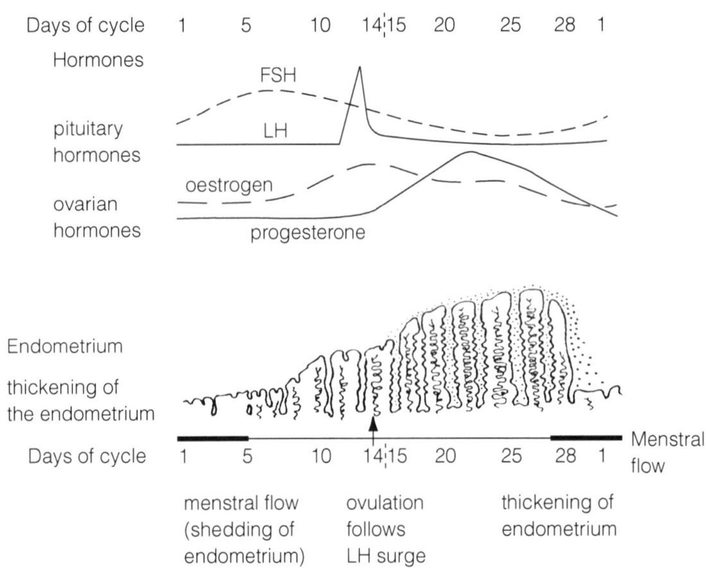

Changes in hormone levels and the endometrium over one menstrual cycle

gland and the cycle begins again. This second two weeks—after ovulation has occurred—is known as the *secretory* or *luteal phase*.

Problems that cause or contribute to infertility

Female factor

Problems with hormones and ovulation

- not ovulating (*anovulation*) or ovulating irregularly (*oligoovulation*)
- polycystic ovarian syndrome (PCOS)
- premature ovarian failure (POF)

- chemotherapy
- ovarian cysts
- advanced age

Problems with the fallopian tubes, uterus and pelvic cavity

- blocked or damaged tubes
- endometriosis
- pelvic inflammatory disease (PID)
- intrauterine fibroids and endometrial polyps
- inflammation, adhesions and Asherman's syndrome
- uterus size and shape and Müllerian duct disorders

Problems with sex

- pain during sex
- vaginismus (difficulty with penetration)

Male factor

Problems with hormones and sperm

- testosterone, GnRH, LH and FSH
- complete absence of semen (*aspermia*)
- complete absence of sperm (*azoospermia*)
- few sperm (*oligospermia*)
- weak or slow moving sperm (*asthenozoospermia*) or malformed sperm (*teratozoospermia*)
- anti-sperm antibodies
- exposure to chemicals
- prescription medications
- chemotherapy and testicular cancer resulting in sperm problems

Problems with the penis, testes and reproductive ducts and glands

- varicocele
- obstructions and blockages

- infections and sexually transmitted diseases
- retrograde ejaculation
- cryptorchidism
- vasectomy and failed vasectomy reversal

Problems with sex

- failure to maintain erection—impotence
- failure to ejaculate
- pain during sex

Female factor infertility

Ovulation problems

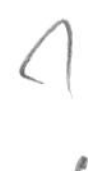

Problems with ovulation are one of the more common causes of infertility in women and, in the absence of any other obvious problem, your doctor will begin by investigating your menstrual cycle. Disruptions to ovulation can be minor and fixed easily, or may be more serious and require more complex treatment. It may be that your ovulation is just a little irregular, or that you ovulate only occasionally—*oligoovulation*—or that you do not ovulate at all—*anovulation*. The effect on your fertility will depend on the cause and extent of the disruption.

Disruptions to the normal pattern of ovulation may be caused by an imbalance of the various reproductive hormones. *Polycystic ovarian syndrome* (PCOS) (see below) is the most common cause of this. Very occasionally, disruption can result from a lack of FSH produced by the pituitary gland due to a lack of GnRH being released from the hypothalamus, a condition known as *hypothalamic anovulation*. Problems may also result from an increase in prolactin produced by the pituitary gland—a condition known as *hyperprolactinaemia*—or from a disruption of the hormones produced by the thyroid. These hormone imbalances can affect the normal development of the follicle and the maturation and release of the egg.

The most common symptom of ovulation problems is irregularities with your periods. Women who have no periods at all, *amenorrhea,* or periods longer than 35 days, *oligomenorrhea,* have an obvious ovulation problem. However, you may still have an ovulation problem if your periods are only sometimes irregular, or even if they are completely regular, although this is less common.

Ovulation induction

Depending on your particular circumstances, it may be possible to induce ovulation with drugs. This is a relatively straightforward treatment involving a short course of *clomiphene* which increases the natural production of FSH and kick-starts your follicles. In some cases your doctor might suggest a low-dose injection of FSH itself which, as long as you are not menopausal, will almost always stimulate follicle development. With both clomiphene and low-dose FSH, the aim is to produce fewer than three follicles. This process can sometimes be a little bit tricky, and it may take a few weeks to successfully induce ovulation.

Once you are ovulating you are monitored by ultrasound scan and may also have a blood test to check your oestrogen levels. When one of these follicles reaches approximately 18 millimetres in diameter, you will be given an injection of HCG to initiate the final maturation and release of the egg. Approximately 24 to 48 hours after this injection is the best time for you to have sex.

Polycystic ovarian syndrome

Many women who have problems with ovulation have *polycystic ovarian syndrome* (PCOS). PCOS is a collection of symptoms that may include multiple small follicles on the ovaries, weight gain, increased facial hair, acne, irregular periods, or occasional periods that are very heavy. PCOS is associated with abnormalities in the way the body metabolises insulin and glucose and, as such, there may also be a link between PCOS and insulin resistant diabetes, especially in older women.

In women who have PCOS, their levels of LH are higher than usual, and their levels of FSH remain constant rather than changing throughout the menstrual cycle. This means that the immature eggs in the follicles fail to mature and, consequently, are not released at ovulation. Also, the relative resistance to insulin is associated with either a rise in the production of *androgens*—the male sex hormones, including testosterone—or an increased sensitivity to these androgens. All women have some androgens, but women who have PCOS sometimes have higher levels. These higher levels interfere with the balance and function of the other hormones. No one is quite sure what causes PCOS; it is often associated with being overweight, but it can also occur in women who are not overweight. It is believed there may also be a genetic link.

Apart from its effect on fertility, overweight women with PCOS have an increased risk of diabetes, high blood pressure, sleep problems and heart disease. With appropriate management, however, these risks can be reduced considerably. Where infertility is the main concern, your specialist is likely to suggest an exercise and weight management program in the first instance. Losing weight may help to restore your hormone balance and periods. This may be followed by treatment with one of a range of medications that regulate the menstrual cycle and induce ovulation. Once your ovulation is restored you have a chance of conceiving naturally.

Some women suffer from polycystic ovaries without the associated problems outlined above. Where this is the case, the condition is referred to as *polycystic ovaries* (PCO), and a distinction is drawn between it and PCOS. PCO is usually diagnosed by ultrasound and may be accompanied by regular or slightly irregular periods. Ovulation may still occur but may not be optimal, and ovulation induction may be appropriate to improve the follicular phase of the cycle. A diagnosis of PCO might prompt your doctor to investigate for PCOS.

Premature ovarian failure

Premature ovarian failure (POF) is where the ovaries produce only a very small number of eggs/follicles, or where the egg/follicle supply is depleted too soon because of a higher than normal rate of egg loss. It can result in either a failure of periods to begin at puberty, or in a gradual decline and disappearance of periods before a woman reaches the age of 40. Premature ovarian failure is also known as *premature menopause* and may be associated with menopause-type symptoms, including hot flushes. There are many causes of POF. It has been associated with auto-immune disorders, pelvic surgery, chemotherapy and family history, but there may also be no obvious reason for it.

Where the supply of eggs runs out completely—that is, there is no ovulation—periods will become irregular and then disappear altogether. Once this happens a woman cannot conceive with her own eggs. Even in this situation, however, there is a very small chance—about 5 per cent—of the ovaries resuming spontaneous activity at some time in the future. Premature ovarian failure cannot be treated with drugs or hormones to induce ovulation because there are no eggs present. The only option for someone with POF is to use donor eggs or embryos (see Chapter 7). Premature ovarian failure is a particularly upsetting diagnosis but it is relatively rare, affecting approximately 1 to 5 per cent of women under 40 who have no periods or do not ovulate.

Chemotherapy

Chemotherapy or radiation treatment can result in primary ovarian failure, or premature menopause. Where this occurs the only real option for a woman wanting to conceive is to use donor eggs or embryos. Technically, it is possible for a woman faced with such treatment to undergo stimulation, harvest eggs, fertilise them with her partner's or a donor's sperm and freeze them for use after the treatment has finished. However, this would involve delaying the chemotherapy or radiation treatment and is therefore not likely to be a realistic option.

Ovarian cysts

Ovarian cysts are small sacs of fluid that develop in or around one or both of the ovaries. They can form from an old follicle that no longer contains an egg, or from an old corpus luteum that failed to dissolve after an earlier cycle. They are usually identified during a transvaginal ultrasound scan. Ovarian cysts are relatively common and, in most cases, they are benign and will have no significant effect on your capacity to conceive.

However, sometimes they can affect the normal functioning of the ovaries, upsetting the hormone balance and temporarily disrupting ovulation. In most cases, they will disappear after a few months of their own accord, but occasionally they can continue to grow. If there is a danger of the cyst rupturing, or if it looks like it might be interfering with your chances of conception in any way, your doctor may suggest you have it surgically removed using a laparoscopy. Once it is removed, ovulation should return to normal. In very rare cases a cyst may be cancerous.

Advanced age

Women are at their most fertile in their early to mid 20s and this begins to decline in their late 20s and early 30s. Fertility drops significantly after 35 and dramatically after 40. This is because, although women continue to produce eggs up to the menopause, the quality of those eggs decreases with age. The longer the eggs are held in the ovaries, the more likely they are to develop chromosomal abnormalities, including Down's syndrome, and the more likely miscarriage is to occur. The uterus continues to function normally and is not affected by age in the same way. In men, sperm function may decline slightly with age, but most men can continue to father a child until well into their 60s and over.

In recent years, age-related decline in fertility has become an issue for many women who, for professional or personal reasons, have chosen to delay starting a family. There is currently nothing the medical profession can do to reverse the effects of aging on eggs. For older women who cannot conceive using their own eggs, the only option is using donated eggs or embryos (see Chapter 7) but, because these are in very short supply, most clinics have an upper age limit on who can access them, though this is not the case if you can provide your own donor eggs. Being older—in your mid to late 30s or early 40s—may not stop you having a baby, but it may make it more difficult. Once you reach 42+ your chances are significantly lower.

One ovary

Women are born with two ovaries that produce and release eggs. Some women, however, lose an ovary as a result of surgery, usually to remove a large or aggressive ovarian cyst. Where an ovary is lost, the one functioning ovary generally takes over the work of both, and starts to produce eggs every month. All else being well, a woman with one functioning ovary has the same chance of conceiving naturally as a woman with two.

Problems with the fallopian tubes or uterus

Blocked or damaged tubes

A blocked or damaged fallopian tube may stop sperm reaching an egg or, if the sperm does manage to get through to the egg, the resulting embryo may not be able to reach the uterus. One or both tubes may be damaged and the damage may occur anywhere along

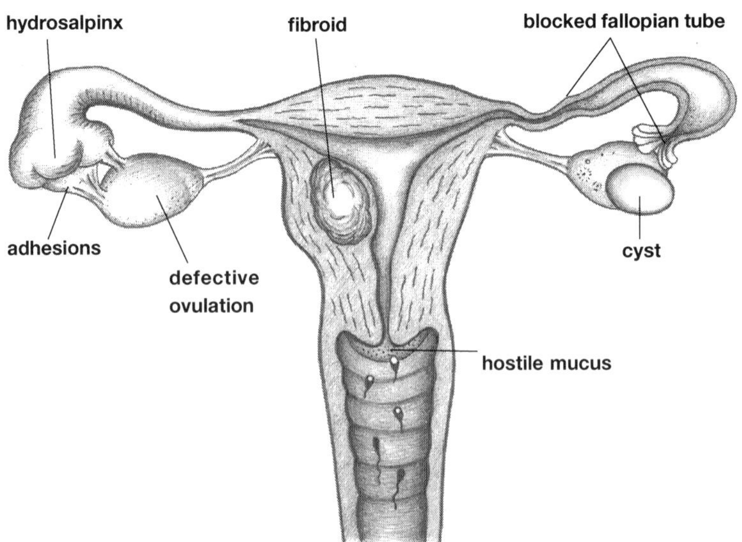

The female reproductive system showing causes of infertility

the tube from the *fimbrial* end—where the eggs enter—to the *isthmus*—the end closest to the uterus. Problems of tubal obstruction are relatively common and, depending on your particular circumstances, there are a range of treatment options. It is this condition that IVF was originally developed to overcome.

Tubes may become blocked in a range of circumstances: because of *salpingitis* (an infection or inflammation), or because of *adhesions* (very thin layers of scar tissue that develop and cause an obstruction), or because of the development of a *hydrosalpinx* (a fluid-filled blockage). In other cases, the tubes may have been cut or tied in previous surgery or, in very rare instances, may have been blocked since birth.

Inflammation of the tube can be caused by infection from sexually transmitted diseases, including *chlamydia* and *gonorrhoea*, from the spread of bacteria from the anus or urethra, or from the insertion of an *intrauterine contraceptive device* (IUD). The symptoms of infection can include pain or soreness, high temperatures and vaginal discharge, but equally there may be no symptoms at all. Where an infection is detected it can be treated with antibiotics and, as long as there is no lasting damage to the tube, natural conception should be possible.

If an infection recurs, or goes untreated, scar tissue may develop and interfere further with the normal functioning of the tubes. The delicate structures inside the tube—the muscle and the little hair-like tentacles that move the egg along, the *cilia*—can become damaged. Sometimes, a blockage in a tube that is damaged along its length can result in the development of a hydrosalpinx, a watery fluid that gathers in the tube and causes it to distend. Hydrosalpinges generally occur at the outer end of the tube near the fimbria and, as such, either stop the egg being picked up in the tube, or stop the sperm reaching it from the other side. It is also possible that, because of changes to the tube caused by fluctuating hormone levels, the watery fluid can suddenly be released and flow down into the uterus, washing away any embryo that may have formed in the other tube.

Where the hydrosalpinx is small and the rest of the tube is okay, your doctor may be able to remove it with surgery. Where this is not possible, they may remove the tube, especially if you have had quite a lot of treatment without success. However, sometimes it is not possible to remove the tube because of the presence of adhesions, in which case your doctor may just clip it to stop any fluid spreading into the uterus.

Problems can also result from adhesions, thin layers of tissue that resemble cling film. The adhesions can surround the ovary or the opening of the tube, and they obstruct the release of the egg or block the path of the sperm. Adhesions can also cause some of the organs and structures of your abdominal or pelvic cavities to become joined where they should remain completely separate—for example, your uterus becomes attached to your bladder. Adhesion may be caused by infection, endometriosis (see below) or previous surgery. Where it is clear that adhesions are interfering with conception, your doctor may suggest removing them by laparoscopic surgery. The problem with removing adhesions, however, is that they can grow back and often do so quite quickly.

The treatment for tubal obstruction will depend on the exact nature of your problem, and it will take into account a range of factors, including whether only one or both tubes are affected, how long you have been trying to get pregnant, what other factors might be contributing to your infertility and your age. Where drug treatment or microsurgery are not appropriate or successful, your doctor may suggest moving onto IVF so that damaged or blocked tubes can be circumvented.

Endometriosis

Endometriosis is a condition where the tissue of the endometrium—the lining of the uterus—grows in other parts of the abdominal or pelvic cavities. It can affect normal ovarian function and, in more serious cases, can cause adhesions which block the fallopian tubes. It can also cause pelvic pain which may result in your having less frequent sex. Endometriosis is believed to occur as a result of menstrual blood or tissue flowing out through the tubes into the abdominal cavity rather than being expelled through the vagina. It is thought some women may have a genetic predisposition towards endometriosis.

Endometriosis is usually detected during an exploratory laparoscopy where your doctor will be able to see small red or brown spots or blisters on other organs or tissue in your abdomen. These spots or blisters can start to bleed, especially at the time of menstruation. The effect of endometriosis on fertility will depend on where the spots or blisters appear and how widespread they are. In more severe cases, this stray tissue may form into a kind of cyst in the ovary called an endometrioma or a 'chocolate' cyst—so called because of the colour and consistency of the thick fluid that develops inside. Endometriomas can restrict the development and release of the eggs from the ovary. Medical experts are less certain, however, about the extent to which mild or moderate endometriosis affects fertility. It is believed there may be a connection between mild endometriosis and problems conceiving, but exactly what happens to cause this, and why, is not clearly understood.

Endometriosis is a reasonably common condition which is thought to affect approximately 20 per cent of all women. It can occur at any age, and may be more likely if there is a family history of the disease. Women with endometriosis may have painful periods, or painful bowel movements, and may experience pain during sex. They may also experience premenstrual spotting or heavy periods. However, you can also have mild endometriosis and have no symptoms at all.

There is a range of treatment options available for endometriosis depending on its nature and severity. If it is present, but there is no associated pain and no obvious impediment to conception, your doctor may choose to leave it alone and just monitor its development. Or your doctor may suggest you have the endometriosis surgically removed with a *laparoscopy* or *laparotomy*. This is generally done by electrocautery—an electric current is passed through a fine surgical needle causing the tissue to evaporate—or by laser surgery or surgical excision. There is evidence to suggest that the more widespread and severe the endometriosis, the more successful removing it will be in improving fertility—as long as all the endometriosis is removed and no significant adhesions form as a result of the surgery.

Pelvic inflammatory disease

Pelvic inflammatory disease (PID) is an inflammation or infection that travels up the vagina through the uterus to the fallopian tubes. It is often caused by sexually transmitted diseases, particularly *gonorrhoea* or *chlamydia*. It can also result from previous surgery, from appendicitis or from an injury to the bowel. It is also associated with the use of *intrauterine contraceptive devices* (IUD). Acute PID is a common cause of tubal fertility problems and is relatively easy to treat with antibiotics, but the effects—or damage—are not so easy to deal with.

Women who have PID may experience more and less severe symptoms depending on the extent of the infection. These can include pain in the abdominal area or pain when urinating, abnormal bleeding or vaginal discharge, a fever or chill. The infection can be treated effectively with antibiotics. If it is not treated it can result in scarring that will further impede fertility. In more severe cases it can block the tubes altogether, or result in the formation of hydrosalpinges (see above). In the majority of cases, however, PID can be dealt with quickly and without recourse to surgery. Once the infection has cleared up, normal conception should be possible.

Intrauterine fibroids and endometrial polyps

A *fibroid* is a benign (non-cancerous) tumour that develops in the uterus. It is sometimes referred to as a *myoma*, so named because it forms on the muscle wall of the uterus—the *myometrium*. A fibroid is usually detected by an ultrasound scan or sonohysterogram, or during an exploratory laparoscopy or hysteroscopy (see Chapter 1). It is not clear exactly what causes fibroids to develop, though they are associated with changes in oestrogen and progesterone levels. Fibroids are reasonably common and are more common in older women.

The effect of a fibroid on your fertility will depend on its size and position—that is, where it is located in the cavity and whether it is interfering with implantation. In most cases, however, it will not be a significant impediment to conception and your doctor will probably just want to monitor it. If it is greater than six or seven centimetres in diametre, and in the uterine wall, it is thought it may cause a diversion in the flow of blood, or cause changes to the hormones, but this is not known for certain.

In some cases, it may be possible to treat a fibroid with drugs that reduce its hormonal stimulation and cause it to shrink. However, though this may be helpful in the short term, the fibroid can often return once the drugs are stopped. Sometimes fibroids can grow to the size of a grapefruit and, where they do, will inevitably

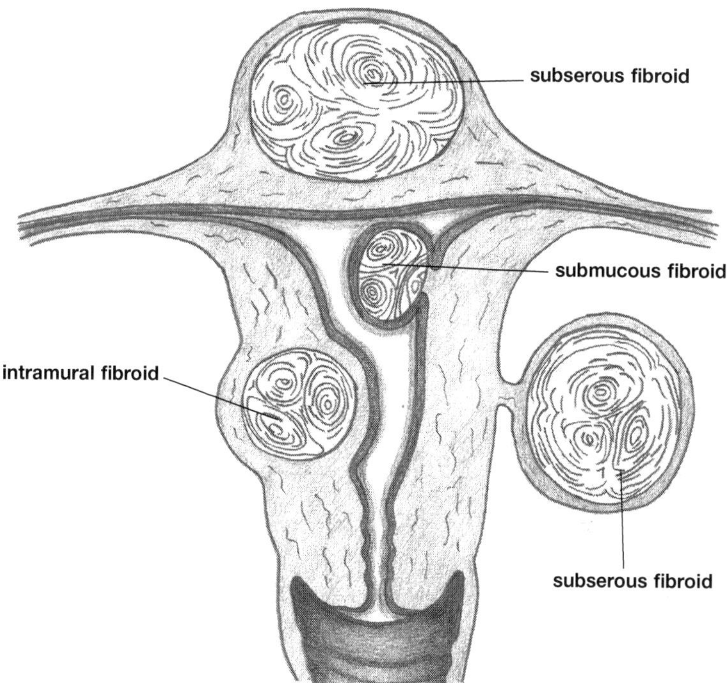

The uterus showing different types of fibroids

interfere with the normal functioning of the uterus. A large fibroid can block the movement of sperm or egg, disrupt the implantation of the embryo, and can cause complications with pregnancy should conception occur.

A fibroid may form on the outside of the uterus (*a subserous fibroid*) within the uterus wall (*an intramural fibroid*), or it may protrude into the cavity of the uterus (*a submucus fibroid*). A subserous fibroid—if it is small and not interfering with fertility—may not need to be removed. If it continues to grow it can sometimes be removed by laparoscopy, but more often by laparotomy or *myomectomy*—the surgical removal of a fibroid/myoma. Submucus fibroids can be dealt with by hysteroscopy. An intramural fibroid is more difficult to remove and usually requires a laparotomy.

Sometimes a benign growth forms on the lining of the endometerium—an endometrial *polyp*. Polyps can cause heavy periods or spotting between periods. They are normally detected with an ultrasound scan and can be treated by hysteroscopy. An endometrial polyp should not significantly interfere with conception.

Inflammation, adhesions and Asherman's syndrome

Inflammation can occur in the uterus as well as the fallopian tubes and can affect the capacity of the uterus to receive and nurture an embryo. An infection of the endometrium, *endometritis* (as opposed to *endometriosis*) can result from *chlamydia* or *ghonorrhoea*, or can occur where there is inflammation that is chronic. In rare cases, the uterine cavity can become blocked with scar tissue/adhesions formed as a result of a previous *currette* (the process used for terminations, or to remove any pregnancy tissue after a miscarriage—what we usually call a 'D&C').

Sometimes the two sides of the uterus can start to grow together causing an obstruction. In more extreme cases this can result in the destruction of the endometrium, a condition known as *Asherman's Syndrome*. Where this occurs conception—even with medical assistance—is highly unlikely, and often surgery is required to restore the cavity.

It is possible to treat an infection with antibiotics and restore the chances of natural conception. Treatment for adhesions is more complex and involves careful, intricate surgery to remove or separate them. Depending on the extent of the adhesions, however, this can be extremely difficult to achieve. Also, because adhesions often grow back after surgery, repeated attempts to surgically remove them may be required. Having intrauterine adhesions will not necessarily stop you getting pregnant but, in the more extreme cases, they can have a significant impact on your fertility.

Uterus size and shape and Müllerian duct disorders

A normal uterus can be a range of slightly different shapes and sizes, and can sit in the abdominal cavity in slightly different positions. None of these normal variations create any problems for fertility. However, there are a number of congenital abnormalities—things you are born with that aren't quite right—and these may have some impact on your capacity to conceive or carry a pregnancy to term.

During embryonic development, the female reproductive organs are formed by the *Müllerian ducts*, which come together to shape the uterus, cervix and upper part of the vagina. Sometimes the Müllerian ducts do not form in a normal way and anatomical anomalies result. Where this happens the problem is often identified at puberty but, if not, it may be uncovered during clinical investigations for infertility. Müllerian duct anomalies are rare, but if they do occur they may have an impact on fertility.

In the most extreme cases the Müllerian ducts fail to develop at all, or fail to join as they should, therefore no uterus is formed. The ovaries may form and function normally—so there is ovulation—but, because there is no uterus, there is no chance of conception. There is no treatment for this condition and a woman with no uterus can never carry a baby. Technically, she could use a surrogate to carry her baby, though this will depend on the legal situation in the state or territory where she lives.

Some women are born with a *septate uterus,* where a barrier (a septum) in the uterus divides it into two. Where the septum is not as big and doesn't divide the uterus fully, it is called subseptate. It is possible to conceive with a septate uterus and successfully carry and deliver a baby. However, a large septum is associated with a slightly higher risk of miscarriage. It is also possible to remove the septum surgically and restore the uterus to normal.

Some women are born with a *bicornuate uterus*, where both the inside and outside of the uterus is divided. It is possible to conceive with a bicornuate uterus but, because the normal shape of the uterus is altered, there is a higher chance of miscarriage or breech birth. It may be possible to correct the problem with surgery, but it is a more major procedure than removing a septum, and usually the risk far outweighs the benefits of surgery.

It is also possible to have a double uterus, *uterus didelphus,* where there are two separate cavities. Normal conception can take place with one uterus making space for the other as the pregnancy develops. Again, because of the change in the shape of the uterus, there is a higher chance of breech birth and of prematurity.

Some women are born with two vaginas and may have either one or two uteruses. Usually one vagina becomes preferred for sex. It is possible to conceive normally with this condition, but you will need to make sure sperm is getting through to the right place. It may be that you are having sex on the side on which you are not ovulating, in which case conception will take twice as long. Apart from having an absent uterus, none of these abnormalities should necessarily stop you conceiving or carrying a baby, but they will need to be considered when deciding on treatment.

Sperm–mucus problems

A few days before ovulation a woman starts to produce vaginal mucus which provides a nurturing environment for the sperm. The mucus should be clear and elastic, similar in look and consistency to raw egg white. Most women are aware of their mucus from feeling a slipperiness when they wipe their vagina with toilet tissue in mid-cycle. This mucus dries up shortly after ovulation. Some women who have had extensive surgical treatment of the cervix may have scarring and/or insufficient mucus production. Where it is thought there might be a sperm–mucus problem your doctor may suggest trying intrauterine insemination (IUI) which bypasses the problem altogether.

Difficulties with sex

Pain during sex

Some women experience pain during sex as a result of some of the conditions outlined above. Where this happens you may end up having sex less often, or not having sex at the right time, consequently reducing your chances of conception. Treatment will depend on the cause of the pain—it's possible that what is actually causing the pain is having a direct effect on fertility. Once the pain is overcome, sex can resume normally.

Vaginismus

Some women suffer from a condition known as *vaginismus,* where the muscles of the vagina spasm or contract making penetration difficult or impossible. This is a very rare condition, however. The first approach in dealing with it is usually counselling. If it cannot be overcome, sperm can be inseminated into the vagina by a procedure known as *intrauterine insemination* (IUI) (see Chapter 4).

Male factor infertility

Problems with hormones and sperm

Testosterone, GnRH, LH and FSH

The same hormones that govern the development of eggs in women are present in men where they govern the development of sperm. If the hypothalamus does not produce the right amount of gonadotrophin releasing hormone (GnRH) the pituitary gland does not produce the right amount of follicle stimulating hormone (FSH) or luteinising hormone (LH). Abnormal levels of FSH will result in a failure of the sperm to develop in the testes, and insufficient LH will affect the production of testosterone, which is needed to help maintain the sperm. Men can also produce too much of the hormone prolactin, which can cause damage to sperm. Irregularities with hormones can be identified through blood tests.

It is not clearly understood what causes these hormone problems and, depending on your particular circumstances, it may be possible to restore the natural hormone balance with a course of drugs. This in turn may result in an increased sperm count and a normal chance of fathering a child naturally. Hormone problems in men are far less common than women; anatomical problems or problems with sperm are more likely to be the cause of infertility.

Absence of semen

Some men produce no semen at all, a condition called *aspermia*. This is when there is no fluid ejaculated at orgasm. Aspermia is associated with problems with the prostate gland and *seminal vesicles*, which are responsible for the production of seminal fluid. A man with aspermia would obviously know about this condition long before the stage of infertility investigations. A complete absence of semen means no sperm and therefore no chance of fathering a child. This condition, however, is extremely rare. The only option for a man with aspermia wanting to have a child is to use donor sperm.

Complete absence of sperm

Some men produce semen that doesn't contain any sperm a condition known as *azoospermia*. This condition is also extremely rare. It occurs where the sperm cells have failed to develop in the testes. It is occasionally associated with a chromosomal abnormality known as *Klinefelters syndrome,* where a man is born with an extra X chromosome. Men with Klinefelters syndrome often have smaller testes, less pubic hair and can be tall with long limbs. Where there is absolutely no sperm (even with very low numbers conception may be possible) there is no chance of fathering a child, and the only option is donor sperm. Sometimes, even in this situation, an occasional sperm may be found in the ejaculate or as a result of a testicular biopsy (see below), then conception may be possible using intracytoplasmic sperm injection (ICSI) and IVF (see Chapter 4).

Sometimes the absence of sperm in the ejaculate may be the result of a blockage (see below) where sperm are actually being produced, but aren't getting through. Occasionally, your doctor may recommend a *vasography,* an x-ray procedure, or a surgical exploration to assess whether there is an obstruction. The obstruction may sometimes be surgically removed at the same time but, more often, a testicular biopsy will be performed.

Few sperm

A more common condition is where sperm are produced, but their numbers are low, *oligospermia*, what we more usually call 'a low sperm count'. It is thought there might be a genetic link to low sperm numbers and it is known that certain environmental pollutants can damage sperm. Chemotherapy treatment for testicular cancer can also cause a low or no sperm count (see below). Sperm make up only a tiny fraction of the semen, so having a smaller amount of ejaculate doesn't necessarily mean there will be fewer sperm. Depending on how low the sperm count is, it may not be possible for a man to father a child naturally. However, recent advances in the treatment of male infertility mean that it is possible for a man who has a very low sperm count to father a child using ICSI and IVF (see Chapter 4).

Weak or slow moving, or malformed sperm

Sperm may be present in the semen but have reduced motility, *asthenozoospermia*; that is, they don't move in a strong forward motion. They may have an abnormal shape, *tetraozoospermia*; that is, there may be irregularities in the head of the sperm affecting their capacity to penetrate the egg, or the mid-piece or tail of the sperm may not be fully developed. Sometimes sperm can clump together rather than swim off individually in pursuit of the egg, a condition known as *agglutination*. Most problems that affect the sperm's capacity to move or penetrate the egg can be overcome with ICSI and IVF. This means that—as with a low sperm count—a man with slow moving or poorly formed sperm may not be able to father a child naturally, but may be able to do so with medical assistance. It is important to remember that 90 per cent of sperm can look abnormal, but it can still result in completely normal fertility.

Anti-sperm antibodies

The body's immune system produces antibodies, chemical substances that help the body to recognise and reject foreign substances and diseases. Sometimes this system breaks down and the antibodies actually attack and reject something they shouldn't. In this case, *anti-sperm antibodies* attach themselves to the sperm and interfere with its capacity to move, to swim through the vaginal mucus and to penetrate the egg.

Anti-sperm antibodies develop as a result of sperm coming into contact with blood. This can occur during surgery to the testes, or during a vasectomy, or as a result of severe local infection or trauma. It is possible to suppress the antibodies with drugs, but this treatment is not particularly successful. More commonly, the treatment involves using IVF and ICSI.

Exposure to chemicals

It is known that certain chemicals found in industrial and household products can affect sperm development and function. Usually, damage occurs only where exposure to these products is frequent or long term. It is also believed that sperm can be damaged by exposure to certain environmental pollutants, though the details of what and how this works is still the subject of much debate.

However, it is generally accepted that men who have frequent close contact with some chemical products may have a higher risk of developing problems with sperm. These chemicals include those in paints—particularly lead, cadmium and mercury—and other heavy metals, including aluminium, copper and selenium. Varnish, solvents, industrial cleaning products, adhesives, inks used in printing, loft insulation materials, fertilizers, particularly nitrates, and pesticides may also cause damage. Radiation is known to cause immediate and lasting harm to sperm (see chemotherapy below).

Prescription medications

Some prescription drugs (see also 'Drugs', Chapter 3) can also affect sperm and may have an effect on libido (sex drive). These include drugs for depression, blood pressure, colitis, ulcers and gastrointestinal problems. In most cases any damage to the sperm is temporary, once you stop using the drug sperm return to normal.

Chemotherapy and testicular cancer

Chemotherapy damages sperm. Sometimes the damage is permanent and there is no chance of producing healthy sperm in the future. Sometimes sperm function returns to normal after the chemotherapy has ceased, but this can take months or years. You should be told of the dangers to your sperm, and to your future fertility, before you begin any treatment. At this time you can provide semen for freezing, which can be stored for a number of years without harm. If, at a later date, you decide you want to father a child your frozen sperm can be thawed and used to fertilise your partner's egg. This can be done through artificial insemination or through IVF and ICSI (see Chapter 4). Either way, even if you no longer produce healthy sperm, with medical assistance, you can still father a child.

Problems with reproductive organs

Varicocele

Varicocele are small varicose veins that develop in the scrotum and can affect the temperature of the testes, which in turn can affect the development of the sperm. Varicocele are normally identified during an initial physical examination by your doctor, or may be detected by an ultrasound scan of the scrotum. Approximately 20 per cent of men have varicocele, most of which are small and do not cause any pain or require any treatment.

It is thought that large varicocele and resultant small testicles—usually on the left side—may have some impact on fertility, and in some instances your doctor may suggest surgery to remove them. This is a relatively straightforward procedure done under general anaesthetic at a clinic or day surgery. The procedure takes a few hours and you may experience some mild pain or discomfort for a couple of days afterwards. However, though it is believed surgery *may* have some impact, doctors are not confident it improves fertility significantly. Depending on your circumstances, there may be other treatment options. Either way, varicocele are not a barrier to fathering a child.

Obstruction and blockages

Sometimes sperm can be produced in the testes and develop normally, but may not find their way into the ejaculate because of an obstruction or blockage. Blockages can occur in the *epididymis*, *vas deferens* or *ejaculatory duct*, the system that transports the sperm. Most commonly these obstructions are caused by inflammation or infection from a sexually transmitted disease, or may be caused by former sterilisation surgery, or they may be congenital. Damage to the vas deferens can sometimes result from a past hernia repair.

A blockage may be detected during a physical examination of the penis and testes, or by vasography—an x-ray procedure done in a day surgery—or may be diagnosed by doing a *testicular biopsy*. A testicular biopsy is done under a local or general anaesthetic. A small amount of tissue is taken from the testes with a needle and examined in a laboratory. This is normally accompanied by a blood test to check levels of FSH which will help the doctor confirm the diagnosis. If the blockage is caused by an infection, it may be treated with antibiotics or, depending on your particular circumstances, your doctor may suggest removing the blockage by microsurgery. Once the blockage has been removed you should have every chance of fathering a child. If the blockage cannot be treated with drugs or surgery it is still

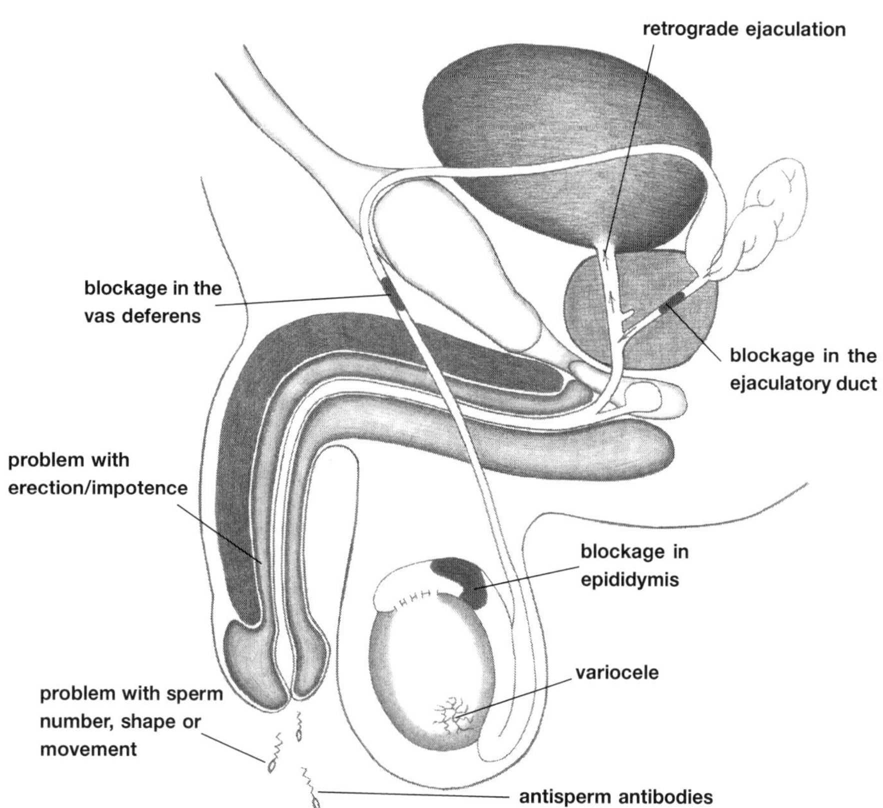

The male reproductive system showing causes of infertility

possible, with medical assistance, to father a child by extracting the sperm through testicular biopsy. The sperm obtained this way can then be used in conjunction with ICSI and IVF.

Some men are born without vas deferens, which means they cannot father a child naturally. This is normally associated with men who carry one of the genetic mutations associated with cystic fibrosis, though they do not actually have cystic fibrosis. It is relatively rare and, as long as sperm are being produced, treatment with testicular biopsy, IVF and ICSI—as with any blockage—can restore the chance of fathering a child. The same goes for men who are born with an abnormal epididymis.

Infections and sexually transmitted diseases

Past or current infections can affect fertility either by damaging sperm directly or by causing an obstruction (see above). Mumps, an infectious disease caused by a virus, in adolescence can cause permanent damage to the testes or impaired sperm development which may leave the adult with no or few functioning sperm. *Prostatitis* (an infection of the prostate), *epididymitis* (an inflammation or infection of the epididymis) and *orchitis* (an inflammation of the testes) can all cause problems for fertility. Infection is normally indicated by a soreness in the testicular area. Most infections can be treated with antibiotics.

A number of sexually transmitted diseases (STDs) can interfere with fertility, including *gonorrhoea*, *chlamydia*, genital warts and genital *herpes*. Symptoms of gonorrhoea and chlamydia include abdominal pain, pain or a burning sensation when urinating, and discharge from the penis. Both gonorrhoea and chlamydia can be treated with antibiotics. Genital warts are caused by a virus; they are quite common and very contagious. They may be treated either with surgery to remove them or with a preparation applied directly to the genital area.

Genital herpes is a viral infection that, once contracted, stays with you. This doesn't mean that you have it all the time, but that it may break out periodically. When you first contract herpes, symptoms can include swollen glands, abdominal pain, sores on the mouth or genitals, and sometimes a fever or flu-type symptoms. Recurring symptoms include an outbreak of sores on the mouth or genitals accompanied by soreness or itching. An ointment may help ease the sores, but there is no other treatment or cure. It is not believed, however, to have any direct effect on fertility.

Retrograde ejaculation

Retrograde ejaculation is where part of the ejaculate moves backwards into the bladder rather than forwards through the urethra and out of the penis. Retrograde ejaculation may be caused by bladder or prostate surgery or by diabetes. It is associated with certain medications for high blood pressure. It can also be a problem for men who have suffered spinal cord injuries or who are paraplegic.

Where retrograde ejaculation occurs sperm sometimes end up being mixed in with urine and expelled during urination. A diagnosis can be made by examining a urine sample—produced after sex or masturbation—for the presence of sperm. Retrograde ejaculation can sometimes be treated with drugs. If this is not possible or effective, however, it is still possible to father a child by retrieving sperm from the urine using specialised techniques, or by using testicular biopsy in conjunction with ICSI and IVF.

Cryptorchidism

Cryptorchidism is a condition where the testes fail to descend into the scrotum as an infant. Normally an operation is performed to correct it, but even where this happens there may still be problems with sperm production and development in the adult. Cryptorchidism can result in oligospermia, few sperm, and may make fathering a child naturally difficult. However, this can be overcome using IVF and ICSI.

Vasectomy

It is possible to reverse the effects of sterilisation, a *vasectomy,* with a *vasovasostomy*, or *vasoepididymostomy*, a surgical procedure that restores the function of the *vas deferens* and enables sperm to be ejaculated. Its success, however, depends on the number of years since the vasectomy was performed—the closer in time the reversal is to the original operation, the better the chance of success. It is also dependant on the presence of anti-sperm antibodies. If there are high numbers of anti-sperm antibodies in the blood, there is less chance of success. Approximately 70 to 80 per cent of reversals performed by trained microsurgeons are successful when performed within about ten years of a vasectomy.

Other blockages, those caused by infection, for example, may also be treated in this way. The procedure is performed under general anaesthetic and you can normally return to work a couple of days afterwards. Approximately six to eight weeks after the procedure, you will start to have monthly semen analyses to assess the quality of your sperm. It can take 18 months to two years for the sperm to return to healthy function.

Difficulties with sex

Impotence or failure to ejaculate

Many men at some time in their lives suffer from impotence—the failure to maintain an erection during sex. It is a relatively common problem that can have a medical, physical or psychological cause. Certain medications are known to contribute to erection problems including tranquilisers, antidepressants and drugs to treat hypertension. Alcohol is also known to have an effect. Psychological issues, however, are the most common cause of impotence. Treatment will depend on the cause, but may include medication, counselling or sexual therapy.

Some men may not be able to ejaculate even though there are no anatomical problems or blockages in the sperm transport ducts. As with impotence, most often the cause is psychological, and treatment can involve counselling or sex therapy.

Pain during sex

This is much less common for men than women, but some of the conditions outlined in this chapter may cause pain during sex, which can result in sex being less frequent, or not happening at the right time for conception. It is also quite possible that the pain is related to something that is having a more direct impact on your fertility.

Treatment will depend on the cause of the pain, but once it has been dealt with, all else being well, you should be able to resume normal sexual activity.

Summing up

By your second or third consultation with an infertility specialist you should have an idea of what's wrong or, at least, have ruled out some things that definitely aren't wrong. Remember, though, approximately 20 to 25 per cent of infertile couples are diagnosed with *idiopathic* infertility—cause or causes unknown. If something specific has been identified, your doctor may suggest a particular treatment, but if not, they may want to investigate further or start you on an IVF cycle. Below is a summary of the preliminary treatments outlined in this chapter, everything up to, but not including, assisted conception and IVF, that might help to resolve your infertility problem:

- drug or hormone treatment to regulate or induce ovulation and restore periods
- weight control to manage polycystic ovarian syndrome, and drug treatment to regulate the menstrual cycle and restore ovulation
- removal of ovarian cysts where they might be affecting fertility
- laparoscopic surgery to remove a blockage or obstruction in the fallopian tube
- drug treatment to suppress endometriosis
- laparoscopic surgery to remove endometriosis or an endometrioma
- antibiotic treatment for an acute infection or inflammation
- surgery to correct a congenital abnormality of the uterus
- lifestyle adjustment—reducing exposure to chemicals or medications
- antibiotic treatment for an infection that may be causing a blockage in the sperm transport system

- surgical removal of an obstruction from any one of the ducts of the sperm transport system
- antibiotic treatment for infection of a sexually transmitted disease
- surgery, or the application of a preparation to remove genital warts
- vasovasostomy—to reverse the effect of sterilisation
- drug treatment or counselling for impotence or problems with ejaculation.

One or more of these responses may be enough to restore fertility and allow you to go home and conceive naturally—you might find yourselves pregnant in the next few months. Where these responses don't work, or if the cause of your problem remains unknown, you may be looking at some form of assisted conception or IVF treatment. This is a big step and needs time and thought and lots of discussion. The next chapter gives you some idea of what you can expect if you head down this road.

4

Assisting conception

Medical treatment of infertility

The options for assisted conception range from the relatively easy and straightforward *artificial insemination* (AI) procedures to the far more complex and invasive *in vitro fertilisation* (IVF). This chapters outlines the various types of artificial insemination (AI), including intrauterine insemination (IUI), and guides you—step by step—through the process of in vitro fertilisation (IVF) and embryo transfer (ET) and describes the different variations of this type of treatment. In the first instance, your doctor should recommend the treatment that has the best chance of success for you with the least risks.

Preparing for treatment

There is normally quite a long time between the decision to do a medically assisted fertility cycle and actually starting the treatment as there are a number of things you need to do before you actually begin. You will have a lengthy consultation with a nurse, where you will go through the treatment in detail, and organise practical things, such as signing consent forms and sorting out how and when you are going to pay for treatment. This lead-in time is also a good opportunity to make a few lifestyle changes, to think about how you are going to manage work, to slow down a bit, spend time with your partner, eat well, exercise, read up on infertility and generally prepare yourself physically and emotionally for treatment.

Seeing a counsellor

All clinics employ a counsellor and most will encourage you to see them before you undergo any kind of medical treatment. In some places, and in some circumstances—where you are using donor *gametes*, for example—it is required by law. The counselling session is a good opportunity for you to find out more about the treatment you are going to undertake, to ask questions, and to discuss any issues that may have arisen since your first consultation. While your doctor will explain your treatment, they will generally not have time to talk in any detail about the bigger, emotional issues of being infertile or undergoing infertility treatment. That's the job of the counsellor.

Everyone has doubts and anxieties, and it's important you are honest about these with the counsellor. The counsellor is not going to report back to your doctor that you really shouldn't be doing this treatment because you're worried, or scared, or because you haven't quite got your head around all that LH, FSH stuff. Counselling is not a test you have to pass, it is a support mechanism to help you through. If you live a long way from the clinic, you can ask to see the counsellor and the nurse on the same day, and get all your paperwork done at the same time. Some clinics have satellite or outlying clinics where you can do this.

Signing consent forms

Before you have any treatment, you will both have to sign legal consent forms that acknowledge you understand what is involved in the treatment and you have been made aware of the risks of the treatment. If you are doing IVF, you will also be asked to specify what you want done with any unused eggs, sperm or embryos—usually this is either disposal or use in research. You will also have to sign written consent to the freezing and storage of your embryos. In some clinics you sign the consents with the counsellor, at others you sign with the doctor or nurse.

Organising payment

You will need to find out exactly how much your treatment cycle is going to cost and how payment is organised. This will vary from clinic to clinic; some will require an up-front payment at the beginning of your treatment, some will allow you to pay later. There is normally a basic charge for the particular treatment cycle you are on, which includes laboratory fees, treatment of sperm, scans, injections, blood tests, pathology fees and the general management of your cycle. You should check exactly what is covered by the fee you are paying.

Medicare has a 'global IVF rebate,' which means it covers most of the costs of consultations, injections, scans, blood tests and pathology lab services for 28 days from the first day of your treatment, and some surgical treatments. There will, of course, still be a significant gap payment. This means, however, that you should make sure you do all your blood tests at the clinic rather than going to a different pathology lab (if you go to a different pathology lab you will have to pay that lab's additional costs). Similarly, if you decide not to do your injections yourself or have them done at your clinic, but go to your local GP instead, you will have to pay for that separately.

In addition to your IVF treatment, you will also have to pay a 'bed fee', or day surgery fee, to the hospital or clinic where you have any surgical treatment. This cost will vary depending on the hospital, and you will not normally be able to claim it on Medicare. You will also have to pay for—and cannot claim on Medicare—any additional drugs you are prescribed, donor sperm, storage of sperm or frozen embryos, and additional technical procedures you have done, including ICSI, assisted hatching or pre-embryo genetic diagnosis. You will also have to pay the professional fees of your anaesthetist, and theatre fees, which you may be able to claim on Medicare.

You will need a current referral from your GP that covers the time of treatment, in order to get your full Medicare entitlements. If you have a health care card you may receive some discount on the overall treatment fee from the clinic, and you may pay a reduced bed fee if treatment is done at a public hospital. You will still have to pay full price for most of the prescription drugs.

How much of this is covered by private health insurance will, of course, depend on the particular cover you have. Most plans have specific policy in relation to pregnancy and to IVF treatment, and you need to clarify with your provider exactly what you are entitled to and when any exclusion periods operate.

Consultation with a nurse

Before you start treatment you and you partner will have to attend a session with a specialist infertility nurse. Your doctor will run through the basic procedures involved in your treatment and give you an idea of the timing of each phase. However, in most clinics, the details of your treatment are arranged and explained by one of the nurses. This meeting can easily take an hour or so and should not be rushed. It is your opportunity to talk through the nitty-gritty of your treatment and clarify anything you don't understand.

The nurse should run through the whole of your proposed treatment cycle, making sure you are clear on exactly what each stage involves. They should explain what drugs you will be taking in what dosages, describe their most common side effects and tell you what to do if you have an adverse reaction to them. They should explain the exact timing of your particular protocol and describe all the procedures involved. They should provide you with a written, day-by-day outline of your treatment that you can take home. They should also teach you and your partner how to give injections.

Artificial insemination

Artificial insemination (AI) is a broad term that refers to a number of different ways of artificially getting sperm to the right place for it to fertilise an egg. The sperm used can be that of the partner or husband, *artificial insemination by husband* (AIH), or that of a donor, *artificial insemination by donor* (AID) or *donor insemination* (DI). Donor sperm may be used in a range of circumstances (see Chapter 7) by both heterosexual couples and by single women and lesbians.

Artificial insemination in general can only be used when the woman does not have blocked or damaged fallopian tubes and if she has no pelvic abnormalities. Your doctor may suggest some form of AI where:

- sperm motility is poor
- there is a sperm–mucus problem or other cervical abnormality
- there is a problem with anti-sperm antibodies
- there is a problem with ejaculation
- the cause of your infertility is unknown.

Intrauterine insemination

Most clinics use a procedure known as *intrauterine insemination* (IUI), a relatively simple and non-invasive first line method of assisted conception. At a specified time before the woman's ovulation, the man is required to attend the clinic and provide a semen sample by masturbation (see Chapter 1). This can be done on the day of the procedure, or done in advance with the sperm frozen for later use.

The semen is taken to a lab where the sperm are removed from the rest of the seminal fluid and subjected to a process called sperm washing. Sperm washing removes excess cells and chemical substances and helps to maximise the sperm's motility and chances of fertilising the egg. Where a donor is being used, the sperm will already be prepared and will need to be thawed in readiness for the procedure.

Once the washing process is complete, the sperm is drawn up into a syringe which is attached to a very fine plastic tube called a *catheter*. The catheter is placed into the woman's cervix with the aid of a speculum and the sperm is inserted into the uterus. It is a relatively quick and easy procedure. Some women find the level of discomfort similar to a pap smear, some find it slightly more painful. Either way, you should be up and about straightaway. You do not have to lie down, or keep your legs up in the air, or avoid walking or running or anything else that you think might cause the sperm to fall out! The sperm is inserted into the uterus and the cervix closes over and protects it, so there is no chance of this occuring.

This process is sometimes—but not always—accompanied by drug treatment for the woman. Close to the start of your cycle, you are given a course of low dose fertility drugs—most often clomiphene, or sometimes injections of FSH—to either regulate your cycle or help you produce more eggs. You have to attend the clinic for a scan to check the size and number of your follicles about two or three days before your ovulation is expected.

When the follicles are the right size—approximately 18–20 millimetres—you may be given an injection which triggers your ovulation, or you may be left to surge naturally. Where you are left to surge naturally, you will be closely monitored to ensure ovulation is not missed. Where you have a trigger injection, you will have the insemination between 24 and 40 hours later. If you have IUI without the drug treatment you still have to have a scan to check your follicle development and establish the right time to do the insemination.

IUI is a safe, straightforward procedure that is a lot less expensive and a lot less invasive than IVF. For many infertile couples it is a good place to start if it is appropriate in your circumstances, and it might even make a welcome change from the pressures of having timed sex. Your doctor may suggest doing a number of IUI cycles, but if you have not conceived after, say, three to four cycles, it might be time to try something else. IUI is certainly an option for unexplained infertility, but it is not the only one. You need to discuss all the options with your doctor and then make a decision about what is best for you.

In vitro fertilisation

Proceeding to IVF is a big step and not everyone who gets to this stage will decide it's for them. Your doctor may suggest IVF if nothing else you've tried has resulted in pregnancy or, if between you and your partner, you have any of the following:

- tubal or other anatomical problems that cannot be fixed
- difficulties with ovulation where medication may result in a significant risk of overstimulation
- inflammation or adhesions that might be interfering with fertility
- an obstruction blocking the sperm
- poor quality sperm, or few sperm
- a previous vasectomy or failed vasectomy reversal
- unexplained infertility.

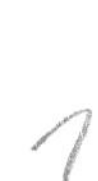

The basic elements of an IVF treatment cycle are the same for everyone, but your treatment may differ from someone else's in a number of ways. There are different methods for managing the first part of your treatment where your natural hormones are suppressed and your ovulation controlled. These are generally referred to as 'protocols'. There are different ways of fertilising the ovum and the embryo can be transferred to the woman at different stages in its development. Dosages of hormones, other drugs used, and the timing of scans and blood tests, will all vary according to individual circumstances. You may also find that different clinics approach the treatment in slightly different ways, and doctors within the same clinic may even do things a little differently. In reality, there are many different courses of treatment, but the fundamentals are the same.

Overview of an IVF treatment cycle

A standard stimulated cycle will start either with you taking the contraceptive pill for three or four weeks before the start of the cycle in which you are going to have treatment, or having a blood test around day 22 to 24 of that cycle to check ovulation has occurred. You then take drugs for a number of days to suppress your own natural hormones. (Depending on the type of cycle you are on, you might take a different sort of drug to control your ovulation later in the process.) You will have a period, then a scan and a blood test to check the drugs are working properly.

You then have daily hormone injections to stimulate your follicles to produce a higher than usual number of eggs. You will have one or more scans during this time to check the development of the follicles and to look at the lining of your uterus. You may also have blood tests to check your hormone levels. When the follicles are approximately 18–20 millimetres you are given an injection to trigger your ovulation. Between 35 to 37 hours after this injection, you will have your eggs retrieved at a day surgery or hospital.

The egg retrieval involves a surgical procedure known as *ovum pick-up* (OPU) or, more commonly, just 'pick-up'. On the same day as your pick-up your husband or partner provides a sample of sperm, usually by masturbation, or your donor sperm will be thawed. Your eggs are passed from the theatre to a lab where they are placed in a culture medium and mixed, or injected, with the sperm. They are then closely monitored over the next few days to see how they fertilise. This is the 'in-vitro' part, meaning 'in glass', referring to the lab dish in which fertilisation takes place (though these days they are actually fertilised in plastic dishes).

Two or three days later you return to the clinic to have one, two or, very rarely, three fertilised embryos transferred into your uterus. Any embryos you do not use can be frozen and used next time, though not everyone will have embryos available for freezing. After the embryo transfer you may be given drugs to help maintain the lining of your uterus to enhance the chances of implantation. Two weeks later you will have a blood test to check if you are pregnant. If you are not, you normally have a break of a month so that your cycle can return to normal.

This whole process—from the first drugs to the pregnancy test result—can take eight to ten weeks. It can be broken down into a series of steps:

- suppression of hormones
- stimulation of follicles and control of ovulation
- surgical egg pick-up and supply of sperm
- fertilisation of the eggs
- transfer of the embryo
- luteal support for implantation.

Learning about injections

IVF treatment involves carefully timed daily injections of follicle stimulating hormone (FSH). These can be administered by a nurse at your clinic at a set time each day, normally first thing in the morning. Most clinics run early appointments for this specific purpose. The injections can also be done, however, by you or your partner at home and, although this might seem a bit daunting, many people find that this is a much better option. If you do them at home you avoid another trip to the clinic so your morning routine is relatively uninterrupted (you can be more confident of getting to work on time) and you can maintain your privacy a little longer if that's important to you. The procedure for giving injections is described below. It should not, in any circumstances, be a substitute for a detailed consultation with an appropriate medical professional.

Your IVF nurse should have a syringe, needles and solvent for you to practise with, and should take you through the whole process of drawing up and administering the injection. It's a really good idea to do a shot in the clinic with the nurse close by to make sure everything goes smoothly. You can practise the drawing up until you feel completely confident, and if there is anything you're not sure about you can ask. The drugs can come in solution, or in powder form, and the injections are drawn up differently. Some clinics have started to use another method of administering the drug known as a 'pen' and it is likely that this will become more widespread in the future. The pen device is easier to use and considered to be less painful.

> I was there for most of the meetings with the specialist and I was there for most of the procedures and I sort of felt intrinsically involved. I mean, I was the one doing most of the injections.
>
> Andrew

Preparing the injection

Stimulation drugs (FSH) in solution

Start by taking the plastic syringe and affixing a drawing up needle to the top. The drawing up needles are generally longer and thicker than the injecting needles and will have a different colour on the wrapping. Remove the little plastic disc from the top of the glass vial of solution and insert the needle into the rubber cap beneath. Gently pull the syringe up making sure all the fluid is drawn into the syringe. The vial contains very slightly more than the amount stated on the label to compensate for any drops that don't make it into the syringe.

Depending on your particular dosage, you may need to use more than one vial. The drug normally comes in quantities of 50, 100, 150 and 200 IU. Ask your clinic to give you the minimum number of vials to make up your dosage. You do not want the volume of the injection to be bigger than necessary, because it takes longer to inject. For example, if you are on 400 IU, it is better to have two 200 IU vials, rather than, say, two 150 IU plus one 100 IU. In the past, problems with the supply has meant this has not always been possible, but it's always worth asking.

When you have drawn up all the drug, withdraw the needle from the vial and—with the syringe pointing upwards and the fluid in the bottom—carefully remove the needle and put in a sharps bin. (If you have not been provided with a sharps bin, an empty glass juice or cordial bottle works well. You must make sure you then dispose of the bottle appropriately—take it to your clinic or to a local pharmacy.) Replace the drawing up needle with an injecting needle, making sure it is secured firmly to the end of the syringe. Remove the cap from the needle and push the plunger in very slowly, forcing the fluid to the top of the needle, but making sure you don't squeeze any out. If you need to you can flick the side of the syringe with your finger to remove any air bubbles. You are not injecting into a vein so you need not be overly concerned about a few air bubbles remaining in the syringe. The injection is now ready to be administered.

Stimulation drugs (FSH) in powder form

The powder comes in a glass vial with another vial containing the solvent with which it has to be mixed. Break the tops of the vials by exerting pressure around the narrow neck and snapping them away from you—or use the little metal file provided to weaken the necks first. Draw the solvent up into the syringe using a drawing-up needle, then squirt it gently into the powder. The powder will dissolve in the solvent and form a clear solution. Depending on your dosage you may need to insert that solution into more powder. The powder normally comes in vials of 37.5, 75 and 150 IU. You can mix two or more powders, of whatever strength, with one vial of solution. When you have drawn up the correct amount, replace the drawing-up needle with an injecting needle. Gently flick the needle with your finger to remove any air bubbles. The injection is now ready to be administered.

More recently FSH has become available in a multidose vial which is easier to use and enables the drug to be administered in smaller volumes. A pre-filled syringe containing water is inserted into a vial of powder through a rubber stopper. The syringe is then withdrawn and replaced with an injection syringe with graduated measurements. The injection syringe can be stored in the fridge and used to administer the drug for several days.

I didn't find the jabs too painful. Afterwards they did sting, but going in it wasn't too bad. I did get knocked around a little bit and I was working full-time so it was pretty stressful. I felt pretty stressed throughout the whole time trying to keep on top of everything. I didn't have much of a social life, but I didn't want much of a social life. I didn't have the energy. My mind was focusing on a lot of other things that were going on at the time.

Tracy

We had all the tests, did the semen analysis and counselling. I went to all the classes, including how to do the injections because I ended up giving Tracy the needles every night. That was fine. Tracy was nervous because she knew I was a bit queasy about that sort of thing, but it really wasn't a problem. I think I did quite a good job actually.

Greg

Giving the injection

The stimulation injections are *subcutaneous*, that is, they go in under the skin. There are three places they can be administered: the stomach, buttock or thigh. If you are having the shot in your stomach you need to sit in a relaxed position so you can pinch the fat on the side of your belly. Your partner should take a sterile swab and wipe the area then slide the whole needle gently all the way into the fat. This can be done straight on or at an angle. Your partner then depresses the plunger, forcing the fluid under the skin and withdraws the needle carefully when all the fluid has been injected.

There shouldn't normally be any blood, but there can sometimes be a few drops. This is nothing to worry about; simply wipe it away with a swab. Try to avoid injecting in exactly the same spot each day, but make sure you are still in the right area. You might find that the injections cause a little yellow bruising, or that occasionally you hit a blood vessel that results in a darkish red or purple bruise. This might look a bit alarming, but is nothing to worry about.

Injections in the buttock go in a specific spot—this is how it was described to me: Draw an imaginary line down the middle of one buttock, then draw another across at the point where the crease separating both buttocks ends below the lower back. The injection should be given in the upper outer quadrant. Make sure the nurse shows you exactly where to do it, and make sure you feel confident about finding the right area each time. You don't have to find an absolute exact spot, but it is important to get it pretty much right. Again, once you've done it the first time, you will find it gets a lot easier. Injection into a thigh is done quite high up and follows the same procedure.

It makes no differences medically whether you have the injection in your stomach, buttock or thigh, and women vary in which they prefer. I've done all of them and will go for the bum every time—sometimes I think it's less painful, or it might just be that

I can't see it! Most women find the hormone injections sting a bit—or more than a bit—and they can be more or less painful on different days for no obvious reason. For your first few injections, you will want to go by the book, but once you get a bit more confident you can try different ways of doing it. If you are having your shots in the buttock you can try it standing up, leaning over the kitchen bench, say, or lying on the bed on your stomach.

Once the needle is inserted the fluid can be injected more or less quickly. As this is the bit that stings I prefer it to be done as quickly as possible, though the instructions tell you to do it slowly. The person giving the injection should be able to feel the amount of resistance and exert the appropriate amount of pressure. If the plunger is depressed too quickly there is a danger of the needle popping off the top. If the plunger is depressed very slowly, you'll be there all day and you won't be very happy. Again, it's just a matter of practice and it really isn't half as scary or difficult as it sounds.

Having an injection is never going to be the most fun way to start your day, but after a week or so you should find it a relatively easy process. A lot of the books say they don't really hurt, but almost everyone I've ever spoken to who has had them says they do—they hurt going in, and sometimes for a little while afterwards too. There were certainly days when the thought of yet another jab made me ill-tempered or teary—or maybe that was the hormones, who knows! Some people really don't mind the jabs and handle them very stoically, others don't. Just remember, you're the one being poked and prodded here, and you're allowed to not like it.

HCG or 'trigger' shot

A HCG shot is given to trigger your ovulation after stimulation. The most commonly used HCG in Australia at the moment comes in powder form. The process for drawing up the injection is the same as for the FSH in powder form. Break the vials, draw up the solution, squirt it into the powder, mix both together, draw the solution

> I think you need to try to go with the flow of your treatment and not expect too much else in your life at the time. Try to have some nice time with your partner and not talk about IVF. Don't expect to have much else going on, don't expect to squeeze things in, because the combination of the emotional and the physical exhaustion is enough.
>
> Tracy

> I used to think I had a very low pain tolerance, but since I've gone through this treatment I actually think I have a very high tolerance.
>
> Wendy

up and replace the needle. The injection is then given in exactly the same way as the stimulation drugs, in either the stomach or buttock.

Other types of injection

Sometimes you may be given diabetes-type needles, which are finer than the usual injecting needles. These can be less painful going in, but it can take longer for the fluid to be injected. Also, each time you insert the needle into the rubber cap, it blunts it ever so slightly. If your dosage requires more than one vial—therefore you have to insert the needle through the rubber cap more than once—you might find that a diabetes needle actually goes in less easily than the standard one. Again, you can try both and see which you prefer.

Some progesterone injections—which may be prescribed for luteal support—have to be administered intra-muscularly and much more slowly because the fluid is thicker and quite viscous. They shouldn't normally hurt, however, even though it's much slower going in than the stimulation drugs. Injections of antagonists—which may be prescribed to control your ovulation in a stimulated cycle—can come as a single needle and syringe unit, and therefore do not have to be drawn up at all.

At first we were quite optimistic, quite confident, I suppose. There was a lot of apprehension too, but we both agreed we would regret it if we didn't give it [IVF treatment] a go. I thought, down the track, I might not be able to live with myself if I hadn't tried. We thought, 'Well, it's available. Let's jump on . . . '.

Tracy

I started off with the nasal spray and the hot flushes and the night sweats—the typical textbook stuff—the raging hormones and headaches. I was trying really hard to remember to do everything, which is where the nurses were so valuable because they'd ring me up with the next instruction. It was a bit terrifying at first.

Tracy

There were no problems with me that we knew of and I was very excited [after the first transfer], very confident it would work. I got loads of eggs and they all fertilised. I was very complacent, cocky even. I was walking around all serene thinking, 'Oh, I'm pregnant'. Then it didn't work. Nothing.

Andrea

I think the only way to do it [go through an IVF treatment cycle] is day by day, because otherwise it's just too much to take in. Even though you can't help looking forward, because you're looking at your dates—when you'll need time off and that sort of thing—you really just need to take it a day at a time. And for the first one, we just did what we were told.

Tracy

Check list of the most common drugs used in IVF

For the purpose of this book, I have chosen not to use brand names in the general discussion of treatment, but to use medical names. I am aware, however, that as patients we often use brand names when talking about infertility drugs, both among ourselves, and with staff at our clinics. Given this, listed below are all the drugs commonly used in infertility treatment with their brand names for ease of reference.

Clomiphene—increases the natural production of follicle stimulating hormone (FSH) and luteinising hormone (LH), which stimulate the ovaries to produce follicles. Taken as a tablet. Most common brands are Clomid and Serophene.

Follicle stimulating hormone (FSH)—stimulates the ovaries to produce more follicles and therefore more eggs. Used in the stimulation phase of down regulated and flare cycles. Administered by subcutaneous injection and, increasingly, by an injection 'pen'. Common brands are Puregon (in solution form) and Gonal F (in powder form and in multidose vial form).

GnRH agonists (nafarelin and leuprolide)—gradually suppress the natural FSH and LH hormones and therefore inhibit ovulation. Used in the suppression phase of a down regulated or flare protocol. Common brands are Synarel ((Nafarelin) nasal spray) and Lucrin ((Leuprolide) subcutaneous injection).

GnRH antagonists—immediately suppress your natural hormones and inhibit ovulation. Used later in the cycle as part of an antagonist protocol. Administered by subcutaneous injection. Common brands are Cetrotide and Orgalutran.

Human chorionic gonadotropin (HCG)—triggers ovulation and provides luteal support. Used in down regulated, flare, antagonist and clomiphene cycles. Administered by subcutaneous or intramuscular injection. Most common brands are Profasi and Pregnyl.

Oestrogen (oestradiol)—enhances the development of the endometrium. Used in artificial thaw cycles. Taken orally as a tablet. Most common brand is Progynova.

Oral contraceptive pill (OCP)—helps the clinic to program your cycle and begins the process of suppressing your natural hormones. Taken orally as a tablet. Most common brand used in conjunction with IVF is Microgynon 20 or 30 ED.

Progestagen—regulates menstrual bleeding. Used to bring on a menstrual period. Taken orally as a tablet. Most common brand is Primolut.

Progesterone—supplements the natural production of progesterone and provides luteal support. Used in some stimulated cycles and with an artificial thaw cycle. Taken either as a vaginal pessary or administered by intramuscular injection. Most common brand of progesterone injection is Proluton.

Starting treatment

Once you have seen the nurse and taken care of all the paperwork and payment, you will be ready to begin. The first cycle can be an anxious, but also a very exciting time—most people feel a mix of apprehension and eagerness. If you've been trying to get pregnant for a while, it can be a real relief to actually get started after all the build-up and preparation. It helps if you have some idea of what to expect, especially for your first cycle, but it's also really important to take each day as it comes. Your clinic should guide you carefully through each stage, and if you have doubts or questions about anything you should always ask. You will find that the more involvement you have with treatment the more confident you will become. At the beginning, when everything is so new and unfamiliar and, when you are having to deal with all the emotional implications of your treatment, you tend to just go along with what everyone tells you. As you become more familiar with the process and the way your clinic manages your treatment, you will find it easier to identify your needs and be more assertive.

This next section describes the process of an IVF treatment cycle in detail; it's pretty complex and technical because that's how the treatment is, and there's really no getting away from that. Don't worry if it doesn't all fall into place first time, or if you get to the end with more questions than answers. That's fine. Write them down and call your clinic. I found the more I learnt about infertility and treatment, the more questions I had. It will help when you read through this section if you concentrate only on the parts that apply to you—at least the first time. If you're not having ICSI or GIFT don't worry about them. You can always look at them later if you're interested. (It might help to refer back to Chapter 3 'How a baby is made'.) Once you actually start treatment, and all this theory becomes practice, it will make a lot more sense.

Your doctor should explain what combination of treatment—or *protocol*—they are proposing to use and why. The standard first line treatment is a stimulated cycle, of which there are two types: a 'long protocol' or 'down regulated cycle', and a 'short protocol' or 'flare cycle'. Both these protocols are aimed at producing a large number of eggs. In a down-regulated cycle there are two phases to the treatment: the first is the suppression phase, and the second is the stimulation phase. Less commonly your doctor may suggest a 'natural cycle', which uses the one egg you naturally produce, or a natural cycle in combination with a clomiphene drug, which aims to produce maybe three or four eggs. There is another, relatively new, protocol likely to become more common in the future, which uses drugs known as *antagonists* (see box). There is no evidence to suggest that any one of these protocols is more likely to result in pregnancy than another; which protocol your doctor recommends will depend on your particular circumstances.

Down regulated cycle or the long protocol

There are two types of down-regulated cycle, usually referred to as 'pill down regulation' and 'day 21 or mid-luteal'. The first part of a pill down regulation cycle is usually, and somewhat ironically, three to four weeks on the oral contraceptive pill (OCP). In some cases you can be on the pill for up to six weeks, depending on the timing of your treatment. Most commonly, a low dose pill of either 20 or 30 micrograms of oestradiol is used, which you start taking on between day 1 and day 5 of your cycle—the cycle before you actually have treatment. The pill enables your doctor to program your treatment more carefully and also begins the process of suppressing your natural hormones. Not all clinics begin with this, but increasingly, clinics are starting this way because of the advantages it offers in the timing and programming of treatment.

Between two and seven days before you stop taking the pill, depending on your doctor's recommendation, you start taking an *agonist* drug, *nafarelin* or *leuprolide* (see box), which suppresses the action of the pituitary gland and stops your natural production of FSH and LH. Suppression with agonists is a gradual process, and you normally take these drugs for somewhere between eight to 15 days. This is the 'down regulated' part, your natural hormones are suppressed in order to ensure you respond appropriately to the hormones that will be injected later. After approximately a week of taking the agonists you stop taking the pill. With this protocol you should expect to have a period around about your normal time, or a little later. You will then have a scan or blood test. If the suppression drugs have done their job there will be no follicle development, and the lining of the uterus will be thin as a result of having a period.

With a mid-luteal cycle you start taking the agonists approximately one week before your next period is due—about day 21 of your cycle—but, because you are not taking the pill, there is no overlap of these drugs. You take the agonists for approximately 12 to 15 days, during which time you should have a period, again around the normal time or a little later. You then have a scan or blood test.

Nafarelin is taken via a nasal spray, usually one sniff each morning and evening for the pill down-regulated, and two sniffs each morning and evening for the mid-luteal cycle, though this may vary depending on your treatment. When you start the FSH, you reduce the dosage of the agonist to one sniff each morning and evening for the mid-luteal cycle and maintain the dosage at one sniff each morning and evening for the pill down regulated. It is not uncommon to experience a range of side effects including, headaches, hot flushes and mood swings. Many women report the nasal spray leaves a bad after-taste in the back of the throat and that, after a while, it can cause irritation around the nose which makes you sniff rather more than usual. Often, women feel tired and lethargic at this time too.

Leuprolide comes in solution and is usually given in daily dosages of 0.1 millilitre with the pill down regulated and 0.2 millilitres with the mid-luteal by subcutaneous injection. The injection is drawn up and administered in the same way as the FSH solution. The side effects are the same as nafarelin, and some women also experience redness or irritation at the injection site. Some women prefer the once only dosage and certainty of the injection, or cannot tolerate the nasal spray.

THE STIMULATION

After you have had a period, and either a scan or blood test or both to check the agonists have done their job, you begin the stimulation phase of the treatment. The aim here is to produce as many follicles on the ovaries as is safely possible. At some time within the next week—depending on how your clinic programs the cycles—you start daily injections of follicle stimulating hormone (FSH). Each morning or evening at around the same time—either at home or at the clinic—you have your injection of FSH. This will cause more follicles than usual to develop so that where you normally have only one follicle you should have a number. How many follicles develop will vary depending on how you react to the drug and also on your age—the older you are, the fewer follicles you are likely to produce. The average number is somewhere between five and 12, although it is possible to produce 20 or more. However, not all these follicles will produce mature eggs, which you need to bear in mind when you are estimating how many you might end up with.

During this stimulation phase you may have one or more scans to check on the development of the follicles and the thickness of the lining of the uterus. Your doctor may increase or decrease your dosage of FSH depending on the size and number of the follicles. You may have an extra day or two of injections and additional scans.

Side effects of stimulation drugs

There are a number of common side effects of the FSH injections, and it is unusual for a woman not to experience something during this stage. The most common side effects are feeling bloated or swollen around the abdomen, mood swings and pre-menstrual symptoms. Other side effects include sore or painful breasts, indigestion, waves of nausea and vomiting, diarrhoea and weight gain. As the days progress you might feel tired and lethargic.

Emotionally, it is not unusual to feel a bit all over the place, and sometimes its difficult to know whether this is because of the hormones, or because of heightened anxiety and anticipation. It doesn't really make much difference what the cause is, but you need to make sure you listen to your body and take care of yourself accordingly. As you approach the time for your trigger injection, you really should start to take things easy. Remember, where you would normally have one 20 millimetre follicle, you could be carrying around ten or 15. Go slowly. Put your feet up. Watch TV or read a book. Make your partner cook dinner and do the dishes.

Ovarian hyperstimulation syndrome

Another, serious side effect that can result from the FSH injections is ovarian hyperstimulation syndrome (OHSS). With OHSS the ovaries are over stimulated, becoming large and painful, and they release fluid into the abdomen. Mild or moderate OHSS occurs in approximately 1 per cent of cases. Early warning signs of OHSS include pelvic or abdominal pain, abdominal swelling, diarrhoea, nausea, vomiting, weight gain and difficulty in breathing. Severe OHSS is rare, occurring in approximately one out of one thousand cases, and it is a very serious condition that requires hospitalisation and a high level of care, including closely supervised bed rest, pain relief, and careful monitoring and management of your fluid levels.

If it looks like there is any danger of OHSS developing, your doctor may reduce your dosage of the stimulation drugs. In most cases, careful monitoring of your follicle development with scans and blood tests will ensure the condition doesn't develop further. It is possible to have some signs of OHSS that will require close monitoring by the clinic, but which may not actually develop into OHSS.

OHSS will almost always resolve itself with your next period. Where OHSS occurs you will not have an embryo transfer, they will be frozen and used next time. You will normally have a break of a couple of months to give your body a chance to settle down and recover. Your doctor will take this into account when recommending future treatment.

MONITORING THE FOLLICLES

After approximately eight or nine days of injections you will have a scan. Your developing follicles should show up on the screen as small dark circles. You should also be able to see the outline of your uterus and the thickening endometrium. Ask the doctor or nurse to show you everything on the monitor and explain what's what. After you've had a few a scans, you should be able to start recognising things yourself. Your doctor or nurse will measure each follicle and make a note of its size, and check that the endometrium is thickening in preparation for receiving the embryo.

TRIGGERING OVULATION

When your largest follicles are at least 18–20 millimetres you are ready for the next stage. Sometimes, if the follicles are not quite big enough, you may need to have another day or two of FSH injections, and a further scan. Once your follicles are ready, you will be told when to have your 'trigger' injection of HCG. Up until now the agonists have ensured you have not ovulated before your follicles were fully stimulated. The trigger injection now overrides the agonist and prompts your ovaries to prepare for ovulation—that is, to release the eggs so they can be picked-up.

HCG mimics the action of luteinising hormone (LH) which is what triggers ovulation, 'the LH surge'. HCG is given by injection either in the buttock or stomach, and may have some side effects, including headaches and moods swings, or may leave you feeling a bit low or irritable. HCG stimulates the eggs to undergo genetic maturation and prepare for release from the follicles. Your egg pick-up is done just before the actual release occurs—that is, less than 40 hours from your LH surge. Injections are usually given about 36 to 38 hours before your pick-up. The time you give the injection is calculated by working backwards from the time your egg pick-up procedure is scheduled. For example, if you are scheduled for a pick-up at 9 o'clock in the morning on Wednesday, you will have the injection at 8 o'clock in the evening of the preceding Monday (37 hours before). You do not need to worry unduly about this as the clinic will calculate your time and let you know exactly when to do the injection. Once you have the trigger shot there are no more drugs for the time being. Now, you are ready for your ovum pick-up (see below).

The flare cycle or short protocol

The other type of stimulated cycle you may begin with is the flare cycle or short protocol. This is recommended less frequently than the down regulated, but is also a first-line treatment option. With this protocol there is less suppression of your natural hormones.

Most clinics begin this protocol with the pill—to help with their progamming— though it can be done without.

You begin taking the pill for three to four weeks immediately before treatment and then have a normal period. On day two of your cycle you start taking the suppression drugs—the agonists—which you take for approximately ten to 14 days. On day three you start the daily FSH injections. The agonists initiate a flare of FSH and LH activity for a couple of days before their suppressing effect kicks in and capitalises on this flare to stimulate your follicles. You normally have the FSH injections for approximately ten to 14 days, and a scan around day 8 to 10. When the largest follicles reach at least 18–20 millimetres you have your trigger shot of HCG and will be booked in for your ovum pick-up. This protocol has the advantage of being shorter than the down regulated cycle and you thus avoid an extra week or two taking the agonists. The disadvantage can be that it doesn't give your doctor quite as much control over your cycle.

Antagonist protocol

There is another type of stimulated cycle which is likely to become more common in the future. On this protocol you do not take any agonists before or during stimulation, but take a different drug—an *antagonist*—later in the cycle to control your ovulation. Antagonists work by immediately suppressing any natural hormones and preventing your ovulation.

This protocol can start with three or four weeks on the pill, though, again, it doesn't necessarily have to. After you have your period—or if have taken the pill, a withdrawal bleed which may be light and short—you begin daily injections of FSH on approximately day three of your cycle. After five to six days of injections you have a scan to check your follicle development. When the largest follicle is approximately 14–16 millimetres you have a blood test to check your hormone levels and begin the injection of antagonist. You may need injections for two, three or four days while your follicles reach maturity. Sometimes a single injection may be available, but this is currently very expensive. You continue taking the antagonist up to and including the day of your HCG trigger shot when you will be given a time for your pick-up.

This protocol has the advantage of avoiding two weeks on the agonists (nafarelin or leuprolide) while still providing good control over your ovulation. The disadvantage is that, at the moment at least, it is more expensive.

Agonists and antagonists

GnRH agonists and GnRH antagonists are synthetic hormones that are closely related to the natural hormone gonadotropin releasing hormone (GnRH) (see Chapter 3). GnRH is produced by the hypothalamus, an area of the brain, to stimulate the pituitary gland, which in turn stimulates the production of FSH and LH. When you start taking agonists (nafarelin and leuprolide) they initially stimulate the pituitary gland to produce FSH and LH, but within a few days start to suppress the release of FSH and LH. This means that the drug you are injecting to stimulate your follicles—the FSH—can do its job without being affected by your natural hormones. Because the LH is being suppressed there is no LH surge to trigger ovulation. It takes a number of days, however, for this suppression to take effect.

GnRH antagonists stop the pituitary gland releasing FSH and LH—and therefore control ovulation—but, unlike agonists, their effect is immediate, which means they can be administered later in the treatment cycle, closer to the time you would normally ovulate.

Natural and clomiphene cycles

Your doctor may recommend a natural or clomiphene cycle if you don't respond well to stimulation, or if you have a religious or ethical objection to freezing embryos, or to creating more embryos than you need. The aim of a natural cycle is to use your own menstrual cycle, picking up the one egg you produce. You do not take any drugs to suppress your natural hormones or to stimulate your follicles. The aim of a clomiphene cycle is to produce two or three eggs by using a low-dose fertility drug.

NATURAL CYCLE

The programming of a natural cycle is based on your usual menstrual cycle. Depending on the length of your cycle, you have a scan somewhere around days 8 to 11 to check that your natural follicle is developing normally, and a blood test to check your hormone levels. Because there is no suppression with this protocol, there is always a risk that you will ovulate naturally and miss the egg pick-up. Your doctor will try to reduce the risk of this happening by monitoring you closely. Depending on the size of your follicle you may have another scan a day or two later, and even another after that. You can easily have two or three scans with a natural cycle, and blood tests daily or every second day. It is possible to produce more than one follicle in a natural cycle (which would normally result in twins) but this is not common. When the follicle measures approximately 16–20 millimetres you have an HCG trigger injection and are scheduled for your pick-up. Because of the danger of natural ovulation your pick-up is done slightly earlier, 35 hours after your trigger injection rather than 37.

This protocol has the advantage of using very few drugs, but has a greater likelihood of being cancelled because of missed ovulation. Also, there is no opportunity to harvest more eggs that could be used in this or another cycle. You may have another scan immediately before your pick-up to check the follicle is still there and you haven't ovulated. In some instances, your doctor may still give you an injection of antagonist if they need to delay ovulation or pick-up.

CLOMIPHENE CYCLE

A clomiphene cycle works in exactly the same way as a natural cycle except that on days two to five of your cycle you start taking clomiphene. Clomiphene is taken in tablet form—normally for five days—and causes the pituitary gland to increase its production of FSH. The level of stimulation, however, is much less than with FSH injections and you are likely to produce no more than three or four follicles. You have a scan on approximately day 7–10 of the cycle to check the development of your follicles. When they reach 16–20 millimetres you will be told when to have your HCG trigger injection and scheduled for your egg pick-up 35 hours afterwards. As with a completely natural cycle, you may have another scan immediately before your pick-up or an injection of antagonist.

> So I had the stimulation and all the drugs and went in for the egg pick-up. When I came out there was a note that said we had 20 eggs which was very exciting. That was another 'over the finish line' sort of thing. We rang back the next day and we're told we'd made 11 embryos. We were very happy. We were very proud of ourselves. We passed several tests on that cycle!
>
> Tracy

Ovum pick-up

Whatever protocol you are on, you will eventually be ready for an *ovum* (or egg) pick-up (OPU). The medical term for this procedure is *ultrasound follicle aspiration.* Most often this procedure is performed first thing in the morning. In preparation you will be told not to eat or drink anything from, say, the previous midnight, and to attend the clinic an hour before your procedure is scheduled. You will be admitted by a nurse, shown where to change, and taken through a series of pre-surgery checks and questions—the same as for a laparoscopy procedure (see Chapter 1) or any other surgery.

The anaesthetist will discuss with you how conscious you want to be for the procedure. Many women choose to be awake for the egg pick-up so they can see their eggs, or *ova*, being retrieved on the monitor. If you choose to remain awake you will be given a sedative to help you relax. Some women feel a pressure in the abdominal area during the procedure and the anaesthetist should be on hand to monitor your level of comfort and administer more sedation if required. Other women prefer to be asleep throughout the procedure, in which case the anaesthetist will administer a general anaesthetic. If you are awake, your partner may be present and can share the experience of seeing the eggs. If you are having a general anaesthetic, partners are not allowed to be present in theatre.

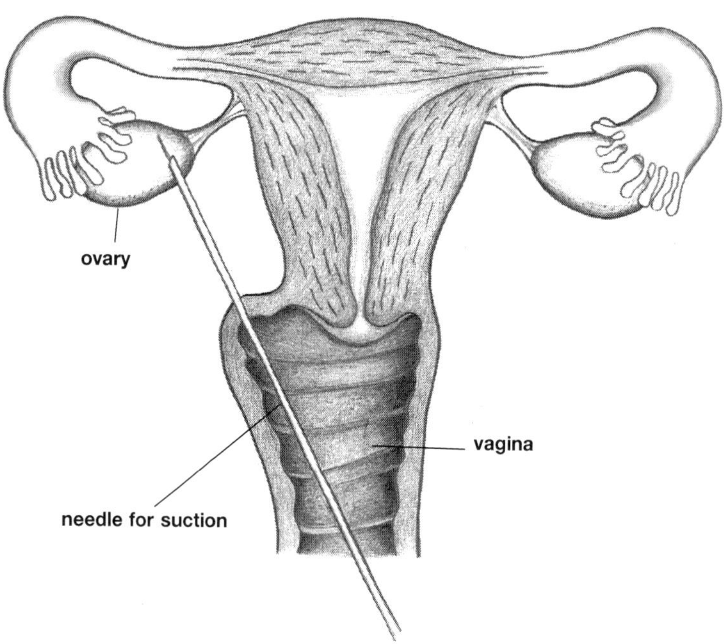

Transvaginal follicle aspiration or 'egg pick-up' procedure

While you are asleep—or watching the monitor—the doctor will insert a vaginal probe with a long thin needle attached. The needle is inserted through the vagina wall into the ovary, using the ultrasound as a guide. This is called *transvaginal follicle aspiration*. The needle is inserted into each follicle in turn and the fluid containing the eggs is sucked out—aspirated—into a tube. The tube is immediately passed to a scientist in a lab nearby who examines the fluid under a microscope to see if any eggs are present. The eggs are then put into tubes of culture medium and placed in an incubator at body temperature. The number of eggs retrieved will vary enormously, but most women can usually expect to have between five and ten eggs harvested, though it is possible to harvest more, but the number may be lower if you are older.

The procedure takes 15 to 30 minutes after which you will be wheeled into the recovery room. You will be given pain relief if required, and the nurse will make sure you are okay to eat and drink. If you had only a light sedative you will normally be ready to go home about one to two hours later. If you had a general anaesthetic you will probably not be ready for two to three hours. The rules about not driving after any surgery apply, even if you only had the sedative, so you will need a lift home. You should be told how many eggs were collected before you leave, and given a number to call for details of your transfer. Different clinics will have different ways of organising this. You may have some vaginal bleeding for the next two to three days and may experience some abdominal cramps for a day or two.

Fertilisation of the eggs

At some stage during the day—normally just before or just after the pick-up—your partner will be required to provide a semen sample. This can be done at home if you live close to the clinic, or can be done at the clinic. The sample will be taken to a lab where the sperm is separated and prepared for fertilising the eggs. If you are using donor sperm it will be thawed by the clinic in readiness.

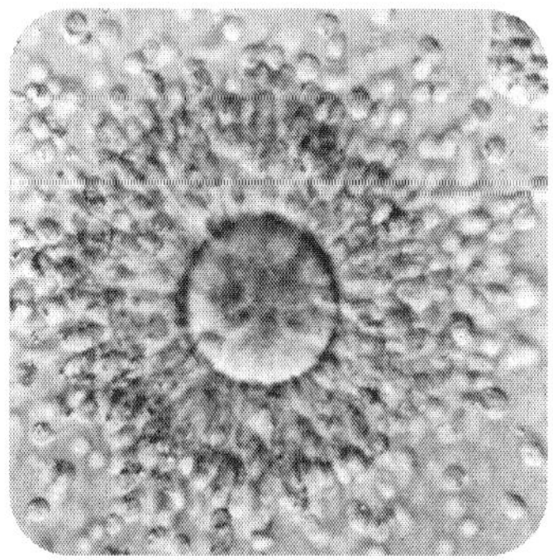

1 human egg (oocyte)

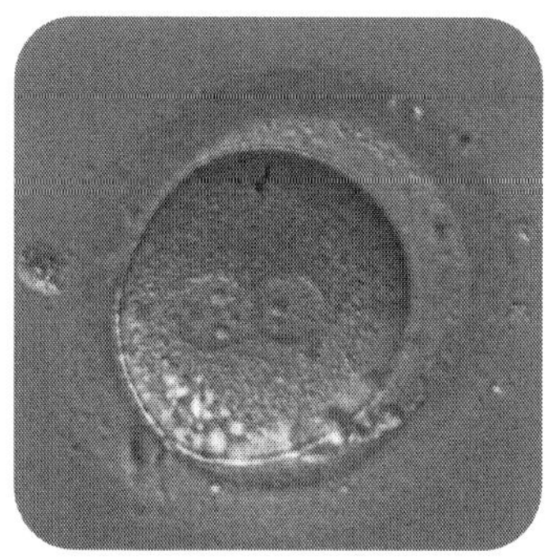

2 fertilised human egg with two pronuclei

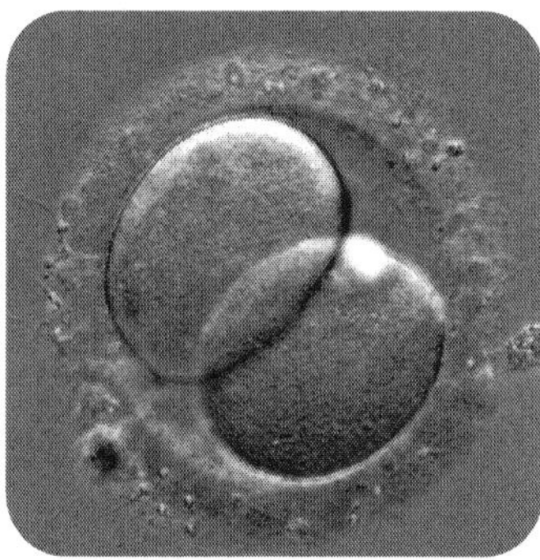

3 two cell human embryo

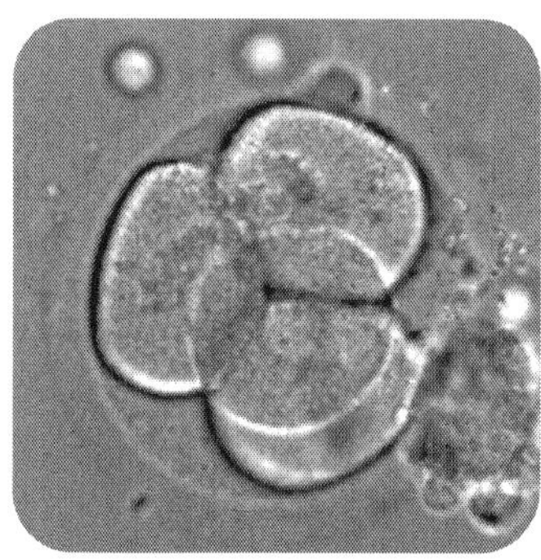

4 human embryo after further cell division

From egg to embryo

The sperm will then be added to the culture medium containing the eggs and placed back in the incubator. Scientists will monitor them at intervals to observe fertilisation.

The individual sperm and egg—referred to as *gametes*—come together to form a fertilised egg known as a *zygote*. The zygote starts to divide and the cells multiply by a process known as *cleavage*. Fifteen to 20 hours or so after fertilisation, two *pronuclei* appear, which the embryologist can see under a microscope. This is the first indication that fertilisation is taking place. Over the next few days the embryo will continue to divide, increasing its number of cells. In most instances an embryo will be transferred on day two or three, but it may be left to develop for a full five days when it becomes a larger, more complex structure known as a *blastocyst*.

Not all your eggs will necessarily fertilise and some that do fertilise may not develop into healthy embryos that can be transferred or frozen. You can expect about a 50 to 60 per cent fertilisation rate of eggs with both IVF and ICSI (see below). In about 5 per cent of IVF cases none of the eggs will fertilise. One of the advantages of fertilising your eggs in vitro is that your doctor can assess your rate of fertilisation and suggest alternative techniques if they are low.

The lab scientists will monitor the development of your embryos. Some clinics will grade the quality of the embryos, based on their size and shape, the number of cells and the extent to which there is any fragmentation (where parts of the embryo have broken off around the edges). The grading system varies considerably between different clinics and if you are interested in finding out more about the quality of your embryos, you should ask your doctor, or speak to one of the scientists. Some clinics do not grade the embryos at all, apart from dividing them between embryos that can be transferred and embryos that won't be transferred.

Intracytoplasmic sperm injection

Your doctor may suggest using *intracytoplasmic sperm injection* (ICSI) where:

- sperm numbers are very low
- the sperm has poor motility
- sperm antibodies are present
- sperm morphology (form) is very abnormal
- fertilisation has not taken place and the reason is unknown.

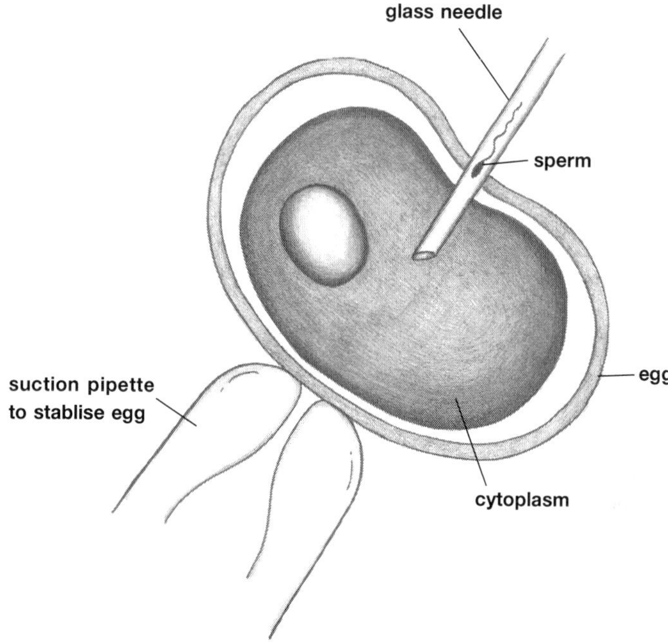

Intracytoplasmic sperm injection (ICSI)

Intracytoplasmic sperm injection—also known as sperm micro-injection—is a relatively recent and very successful treatment for male infertility. It is used in conjunction with IVF and embryo transfer. It involves a single sperm being injected directly into an egg with the use of a powerful microscope. The egg is held in place in a dish, and a glass pipette containing the sperm is gently forced through the *zona pellucida*—the tough outer shell of the egg. The sperm is then injected into the centre of the egg, the *cytoplasm*, and the pipette is then withdrawn.

ICSI overcomes a range of problems where the sperm either cannot reach, or cannot penetrate the egg. Fertilisation rates with ICSI are good, and babies born as a result of ICSI are no different

> My sperm was okay—about average. They said they could pick out some good ones! Our specialist recommended ICSI and we decided to go with that because of our age—we were 38 and 39. We knew it was going to cost a lot anyway so we thought why not go with the most proven method.
>
> Greg

from those born through the conventional IVF methods. ICSI is not included in the normal cost of a cycle of IVF treatment, however, and is not currently covered by Medicare.

Sperm aspiration techniques

In the majority of cases of assisted conception using the husband or partner's sperm, the sperm sample will be provided by masturbation. However, where sperm is being produced but there is a problem with ejaculation, or where the sperm is not reaching the ejaculate because of a blockage or absent duct, or where there is an impairment of sperm production so that very little sperm is produced or not found in the ejaculate, the sperm can be obtained directly from the man's *testes* or *epididymis* by a number of different techniques. Whether the sperm is extracted from the testicles or the epididymis will depend on the cause of the problem.

The most common of these techniques is testicular biopsy which can be performed using a local anaesthetic—where you are awake—or a general anaesthetic—where you are asleep. Sperm are aspirated, or sucked out using a needle inserted into the testicle via the skin of the scrotum. The procedure can cause some swelling that clears up after a few days.

Depending on your particular circumstances, your doctor may suggest aspirating sperm directly from the epididymis. This may be appropriate, for example, where a vasectomy reversal has not been successful. This procedure is performed while you are awake, using a local anaesthetic and pain relief. A needle is inserted directly into the epidydimis and the fluid containing sperm is aspirated.

Embryo transfer (ET)

The next stage of treatment is the transfer of the embryo into the uterus. This is usually done two to five days after fertilsation. You will be asked to call the clinic at a specified time to find out how many of your eggs fertilised and the time of your transfer. In most cases your doctor will recommend one or two embryos be transferred. Very occasionally—where repeated cycles have failed, or where the woman is of advanced age—your doctor may suggest transferring three. Increasingly, however, clinics are trying to limit the numbers of embryos transferred to reduce the risk of multiple pregnancies. The more embryos transferred, the higher the chance of conceiving, but this has to be balanced against the increased chance of multiple births.

Certainly, lots of people who have two or three embryos transferred end up with only one baby, but some end up with twins or triplets. This might seem like a lovely idea—all your babies in one go and no more treatment—but it has to be balanced against the increased medical risks to you and your multiple babies, and the enormous emotional, physical and financial demands of caring for two or, especially, three babies. The bottom line is, if you transfer more than one embryo, you must be prepared for more than one baby. Make sure you discuss all these implications with your doctor and your partner well before any decisions are made.

The procedure

The *embryo transfer* (ET) is a relatively quick and easy procedure that should take no more than a few minutes. For most women it is an uncomfortable, but not painful, experience. In some circumstances, where the shape of your cervix or uterus makes inserting the *catheter* difficult, it can take a little longer and be painful. Where this is the case you can have a mild sedative to help you relax. The procedure shouldn't be painful, but if it hurts you don't have to stoically grin and bear it, tell the doctor. If it is very painful, or if the doctor has real problems performing the transfer, it can be done under a general anaesthetic.

You will be asked to lie on the bed with your legs apart and your feet supported. Often the doctor will show you your embryos on the screen. The doctor will insert a speculum into your vagina, just like a pap smear. Specula come in different sizes and if the one your doctor uses feels more uncomfortable than usual, ask them to swap it for a smaller one. They then insert the catheter through your cervix and into your uterus. When the catheter is in position the embryologist passes your embryos to the doctor in a thin tube attached to a syringe. The doctor—or in some clinics, the embryologist—inserts the tube into the catheter and squeezes the syringe to insert the embryos. They then give the syringe and tube back to the embryologist who checks it under the microscope to make sure the embryos have been inserted. The doctor then removes the speculum and the procedure is over. As with *intrauterine insemination* (IUI), you do not have to stay lying down after the transfer; you can continue your normal daily routine pretty much straightaway.

Gamete intrafallopian transfer

Gamete intrafallopian transfer (GIFT) is a transfer procedure that is performed at the same time as the pick-up. It is mostly used for couples with a religious or moral objection to fertilisation outside the body. At least one fully functioning fallopian tube is required as well as healthy, motile sperm. GIFT is performed in conjunction with a stimulated cycle, and can be used with either a down regulated, flare or antagonist protocol.

The pick-up for GIFT is done in exactly the same way as an IVF procedure. The eggs are retrieved and passed immediately to the embryologist in the lab. The embryologist mixes one or two eggs with the sperm and immediately passes them back to the doctor, who inserts them directly into the fallopian tube using a laparascope. This means that both sperm and eggs are in the right place at the right time and have a chance of fertilising naturally inside the body. The remaining eggs can be fertilised and frozen, unless there are specific religious objections.

Although GIFT can be done in one surgical procedure, the use of laparoscopy makes it more invasive, so you will require more recovery time than if you had undergone the standard ultrasound follicle aspiration and embryo transfer.

> Those last two weeks after the transfer, yeah, they're pretty horrendous. I remember I really didn't want to do anything. My boobs were sore and I'm thinking maybe I'm pregnant, maybe I am. But then I got my period just before the blood test. That's how it seemed to happen with all my cycles. But I remember I was so excited that first time, because we knew someone where it had happened first time, and I thought it would for us. I was pretty devastated, but I thought, 'Bad luck. We'll try again'. Which we did and the same thing happened the next time.
>
> Tracy

Luteal support

Once you have had your transfer you go home and start the long two-week wait. At this point you have one or more fertilised eggs floating around your uterus which now have to implant into the lining—the *endometruim*—in order for a pregnancy to occur. Your doctor may provide you with some luteal support to help maintain the lining as long as possible, and to give your embryos the best chance of implanting. Luteal support may be in the form of *HCG* or *progesterone* (in the form of a pessary or injection—a progesterone gel may soon be available).

HCG is the hormone given to trigger ovulation prior to your pick-up (see above). Your doctor may sometimes suggest you have a further two or three injections of this at intervals of a few days apart to help stimulate your progesterone production. The usual dosage is 2000 iu (international units). It comes in powder form and is injected *subcutanously* in the stomach, buttock or thigh.

Alternatively, you may be prescribed progesterone pessaries. These come in the form of a soft waxy tablet, about 2 centimetres long, that is either wrapped in foil or enclosed in a small plastic capsule. They must be kept in the fridge. You remove the foil or capsule and insert the pessary into the vagina, just like you would a tampon. The pessary melts slowly and the progesterone is absorbed. Most people insert them at bedtime. There is sometimes a little leakage which can be taken care of with a panty liner.

The number of pessaries prescribed can vary from one to two a day, and you continue to take them for at least 14 days, or until you are advised to stop. It is possible that your period will be delayed as a result of using the pessaries, because the pessaries are artificially maintaining your endometrium. You need to bear in mind that a delay in your period arriving might be due to the pessaries, rather than to a pregnancy.

Progesterone luteal support can also be given by an injection, which comes in a liquid form and is given intramuscularly in the buttock. The solution is thick and viscous and cannot be injected quickly. You will find it takes much longer to inject this than the FSH solution, but it should not be painful. It is usually given every second day until you know you are not pregnant.

Where things can go wrong

In this hugely complex process things sometimes go wrong. Often this is not anyone's fault; it's just the way it is. You may not respond to the suppression drugs adequately, the stimulation may not result in many mature eggs, you may not ovulate or your ovulation might be missed, you might suffer from mild ovarian hyperstimulation syndrome, your eggs may not fertilise or they may fertilise but not divide, your endometrium may not thicken sufficiently, your eggs might not survive or might not survive thawing. Any of these might result in a cancelled pick-up or transfer. Remarkably, however, often this complicated, technical process all goes according to plan, and a little miracle happens.

I was pregnant and I was absolutely shocked and unprepared for it—after all this preparation I was unprepared.

Darcy

The two-week waiting period after a transfer is excruciating. I don't think about it too much until about ten or eleven days afterwards. That's when I start thinking maybe? And the clinic tell you every time, you know, that you shouldn't use those home testing kits, but you've got to have some control, really. For me, testing at home is about taking back a bit of control.

Wendy

It was the first time I didn't do a home pregnancy test. I swore I couldn't bear to see a negative test again. I couldn't stomach it. After I got the call to say I was pregnant I ran across the road to the chemist. I thought, I've got to get a home pregnancy test, because I've got to see what it looks like when it works. The first thing I did when I got home was pee on a stick and I saw the double blue line. I was at the point that I thought those tests didn't work at all, that it was just a bit of cardboard in there.

Andrea

For the last cycle I almost got to the stage of trying to forget about it, because the one before was so devastating. I didn't want to go through that again, so we sort of basically tried to put it out of our minds. And then it was phone call day and Tracy still hadn't had her period which was the first time. And then I couldn't believe it when I got the news. I was lying in bed reading the paper and the phone rang and . . . I couldn't believe it actually. It was amazing. I was expecting the 'Oh no. It didn't work again', sort of thing. It was a shock. A really good shock.

Greg

After you've had the embryos inserted there's really nothing you can do for the next two weeks until you get the news. So a couple of times when it was consuming us we thought we'd go away for the weekend, go fishing, go to the beach. Do something.

Greg

One thing I do remember about the call was that, because it was such a process and you rely on the clinic to tell you what to do at each step, when they said that I was pregnant, I said, 'Oh okay. What do I do now?' Again I was expecting them to instruct me in the next part of the process. And then there's this kind of separation anxiety from the IVF clinic when they say they don't need to see you again. It's like, 'Thanks and see you later'.

Greg

Pregnancy tests

You will be scheduled for a blood test approximately 14 to 17 days after your transfer. The test for pregnancy is sometimes called a beta test, and sometimes an HCG test. Many women say the lead up to the test is the worst part of the whole treatment cycle. The temptation to look for signs of pregnancy at this stage is enormous, but there really are no reliable signs this early. That is not to say, however, that some women might not feel completely confident they are pregnant.

The problem is that the signs of being pregnant are the same as the signs of a period about to start: sore breasts, twinges or cramps in the abdomen, or feeling tired. These could all mean something or nothing. Other 'signs' might just be a result of the treatment. It is very common, for example, for the timing of your period to be affected by the drugs, especially if you've had progesterone pessaries or injections. Your body might feel different in any number of ways that could be attributed to pregnancy, but might just as easily be the result of treatment. It is completely natural to look for signs, and many women find it hard not to do so. Just be a little wary, however, that there are a lot of factors involved here.

The other temptation that is hard to resist is to do your own pregnancy test at home with a kit bought from a chemist. Most IVF clinics advise against this but, again, many women do them anyway. Most over-the-counter pregnancy testing kits work in the same way. You insert a small plastic stick into the flow of your urine first thing in the morning, after your last missed period—different kits are designed for use on different days. You then leave the stick for a specified number of minutes—depending on the type of test—and see whether a line appears indicating a positive result.

The tests claim to be very accurate, but they can vary enormously. Also, the drugs used in your treatment can affect the test result, sometimes leading to an incorrect result. Your HCG level could be artificially elevated, for example, if you have had post-transfer injections of HCG for luteal support. This is why clinics do not recommend them. There are certainly cases of women testing negative with an over-the-counter kit who turn out to be pregnant, and cases of women testing positive who turn out not to be pregnant.

I always did a test at home because if the result was going to be negative I wanted to find out first, at home and with my partner, rather than hearing it from a stranger over the phone. I suppose I then felt a bit more prepared for the bad news. You have to have a blood test at the clinic anyway, so it's really just a matter of timing. Again, it's up to you and your partner. If you do more than one cycle, you can try it different ways and see what suits you best.

The definitive test is the blood test you will have at the clinic. A positive result is indicated by an increased level of HCG, but clinics vary in how they define a positive result. More than 5 iu (international units) may indicate there has been implantation, but most clinics use a level of more than 50 or more than 80 iu to indicate a positive result. It will also depend on what day you have the test done. A level of more than 100 iu 14 days after transfer is a good indication that a pregnancy is likely, but it may also be likely if the level is somewhat lower less than this.

Your clinic may suggest you have a second test a few days or a week after the first to confirm the result if the initial level is a bit low or if you have a history of ectopic pregnancy (see Chapter 5)—or they may suggest it routinely. Your HCG level should double every two to three days, for about eight to ten weeks so if the pregnancy is viable your levels should increase quite noticeably in that first week. A repeat test allows the clinic to know whether your levels are rising or falling, which gives you a much better idea of the likelihood of the pregnancy continuing.

Test result

Eventually you will make the dreaded call to the clinic—or they will call you—for the result of your test. If it is positive, and the pregnancy continues successfully, you will be thrilled. You can put this book in the bottom drawer, forget about it, and concentrate on enjoying the next nine months. If your test is negative, you might be anything from disappointed to devastated. However you feel, you'll need to give yourself some time and space to deal with your loss (see Chapter 9). When you're feeling up to it, you can call your doctor for another appointment, if you are going to try again. It's also possible that you get a positive pregnancy test result that doesn't, in the end, result in a pregnancy (see Chapter 5), in which case you will want to see your specialist again to decide how to proceed from here.

A period or bleed and a positive pregnancy test

It is possible to have a period and be pregnant. It is not common to have a full period, but it is not unusual to have some light bleeding or spotting. While the arrival of a period is a reasonable indicator that you are not pregnant, it does not necessarily mean that you aren't. If you've had a bleed, often the last thing you want to do is go for a pregnancy test and listen to someone on the phone telling you what you already know. However, because it is possible to have some form of period and still be pregnant, clinics insist you have a pregnancy test. It's important to have it, and it's important you ring up for the result.

Summing up

If preliminary treatments have not been successful, or are not appropriate in your circumstances, you may proceed to some form of assisted conception. This can include anything from relatively straightforward artificial insemination procedures to the more complex in-vitro fertilsation.

A common first-line method of assisted conception is intrauterine insemination (IUI) which may be performed with your partner's or donor sperm, and may or may not be accompanied by drug treatment for the woman. Alternatively, you may proceed to some form of IVF treatment in response to a range of specific fertility problems, or where the cause of your infertility is unknown. The details of an IVF treatment cycle vary between couples, but the essential elements are the same.

- You usually begin by having a number of consultations with an infertility specialist, a lengthy consultation with a nurse and, in some cases, a counsellor. You have to sign consent forms and organise payment.
- In most clinics you start by taking a course of oral contraceptive pill which allows the clinic to program your treatment.
- The first part of your treatment involves suppressing your natural hormones with drugs, and monitoring this with blood tests and ultrasound scans.
- Once your natural hormones have been suppressed you have a series of injections to stimulate your follicles to produce multiple eggs.
- At a specific time you undergo a minor surgical procedure commonly referred to as 'egg pick-up' to retrieve your eggs.
- Your eggs are then placed with the sperm, or the sperm is injected into the eggs, and fertilisation is monitored closely over the next few days.
- At the appropriate time one or two embryos are transferred to your uterus using a speculum and catheter. Any unused embryos are frozen and can be used next time.
- Approximately 14–17 days after your embryo transfer you have a blood test to check your levels of HCG and determine whether a pregnancy has occurred.
- This may be a challenging time for you, dealing with both the physical and emotional effects of the treatment.

5

The loss of a pregnancy

Causes of miscarriage

About 20 per cent of all pregnancies result in miscarriage, irrespective of the way the prenancy is achieved. Almost all miscarriages happen in the first trimester, and many in the first few weeks after conception. Early miscarriage often occurs because there is something wrong with the embryo; it is no more than nature's way of screening out embryos that are not going to produce healthy babies. Because miscarriage is so common, having one or two in a row is generally considered to be in the range of normal—more a case of bad luck than any indication that something might be seriously wrong. Many people who have a miscarriage go on to have a healthy pregnancy the next time without any medical intervention.

Just because miscarriage is common, however, doesn't make it an easy thing to experience, and it doesn't mean that it won't have a significant effect upon you emotionally. Miscarriage always brings with it an enormous sense of loss. Even in the very early stages of pregnancy—especially if you've seen a sac or heartbeat on an ultrasound—you may feel bonded with your baby; even though it is only days or weeks old, you may love it already—many women do. For you, the loss is real and tangible, a potential life inside you that died, a much wanted son or daughter who couldn't stay. It is important you acknowledge this sense of loss and give yourself the time and opportunity to grieve in whatever way feels right for you (see Chapter 9).

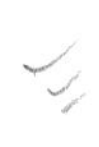

Your sense of loss may be compounded if you've had to wait a long time for your pregnancy, or if it was difficult to achieve, or if it has happened more than once. If you conceive after IVF, a miscarriage can be enormously difficult because of all the emotional and physical energy that has been invested in achieving the pregnancy. Miscarriage after IVF also means facing another round of treatment, just when you thought you would be leaving that all behind and moving on.

> I was just flooding with blood. I had never had anything like it. The doctor confirmed the pregnancy and said this could be a miscarriage or it could just be spotting. It is the most weird word that, 'spotting'. It just doesn't match with this flow of blood. I didn't have any cramps—it was kind of strange—just this flood. They said the usual thing, that one in four women suffer miscarriages and it is usually a good thing if you miscarry, you know, if the embryo was a bit dodgy it is nature's way of getting rid of it. After the second one they said maybe I had been a bit unlucky.
>
> Lee

Early pregnancy loss

Implantation occurs approximately seven days after fertilisation, at which point the pregnancy hormone HCG starts to be produced by the body. At approximately six or seven days after implantation (14 days after fertilisation), raised HCG levels can be detected in a blood

We got pregnant really quickly. It happened in that eager, ego-massaging, confirming way of this is how it should be. It was fantastic. I'm healthy. You're healthy. It was a lovely little thing. Straightaway. We went through the excitement of all that, until ten weeks. Then we had an ultrasound because there was bleeding and things didn't seem right. And then it started to get scary and sad.

Mark

By twelve weeks it was all over. We didn't know why. Things happen. The doctors said, 'We don't know. We can't tell you why.' I thought, 'These things happen'. Lee was more wanting to know why. All that was sort of irrelevant, for me. It hit hard. It was a really major blow. It was probably the only time I've seen Lee—a thoroughly formidable and competent person—knocked down by something.

Mark

or urine sample. This is known as a *biochemical pregnancy* because the only evidence of it is the HCG test. It is possible to have a positive pregnancy test result approximately two to three weeks after ovulation, but for the pregnancy not to continue any further. Where this happens, you may have a bleed soon afterwards so that it may appear as if you have had a late period. In this situation a second pregnancy test a week after the first may have shown your levels of HCG declining, or that there was no HCG at all.

A clinical pregnancy is diagnosed by a positive HCG test and when, at around six weeks, you can see the start of a sac developing on an ultrasound scan. At about six to six-and-half weeks, you would also expect to see a heartbeat. If at any time from about seven weeks onwards there is still a sac and evidence of the foetus, but no heartbeat, you are said to have had a *missed abortion*. If there is a sac, but no evidence of the foetus, you are said to have had a *blighted ovum* (no awards for the terminology). More commonly, these are now referred to as 'early failed pregnancy'. In both these cases you may pass the *products of conception*—the foetus and sac—naturally, or you may be required to go to hospital for a *dilation* and *curette*—or D & C as it is traditionally known. A D & C is a surgical procedure performed under anaesthetic, where a doctor removes any pregnancy tissue that may be remaining. If during an ultrasound scan it is clear that you have passed all the pregnancy tissue, you are said to have had a *complete abortion* (or now more usually—and more acceptably—a *complete miscarriage*) and a curette is not required. If you have had a bleed, but a scan shows some tissue still remaining, you are said to have had an *incomplete abortion* (again these days more usually called an *incomplete miscarriage*) and will need to have a curette. Increasingly, gynaecologists are using medical, rather than surgical, curretage using misoprostol, a vaginally or orally taken prostaglandin. This avoids admission to hospital, general anaesthetics and a surgical procedure.

The most common signs of miscarriage are bleeding—which can be light and occasional, or heavy and persistent—and abdominal pain, cramps, or pain in the lower back. It can also be associated with the disappearance of your pregnancy symptoms: the nausea, tiredness and sore breasts.

Ectopic pregnancy

An ectopic pregnancy is where the embryo implants somewhere other than the uterus, usually in the fallopian tube. Where the pregnancy is ectopic, you will have a positive HCG test—because pregnancy hormones are still being produced—but there will be no pregnancy in the uterus. Further investigation with ultrasound will show evidence of the pregnancy forming in the fallopian tube or elsewhere. If HCG levels are greater than 1200 iu, it would be expected to see a pregnancy sac inside the uterus. Failure to see a sac would suggest ectopic pregnancy and the need for laparoscopy. Lower HCG levels may suggest an early healthy pregnancy, an early failing pregnancy or ectopic pregnancy. Repeated tests for HCG levels and scans may be required to identify exactly where the pregnancy is forming.

Ectopic pregnancies occur in approximately 3–4 per cent of pregnancies and you have a slightly increased chance of having an ectopic pregnancy if you have pre-existing tubal disease. The causes of ectopic pregnancy are not clearly known, but they are associated with damage to the tubes from infection or previous surgery, and with some hormone disturbances, though they can still occur where none of these are present.

Symptoms of ectopic pregnancy include discomfort and pain in the lower abdominal area, which may be to one side. Bleeding is also common and this may be different from your usual period; it can be less heavy or darker in colour. The bleeding may continue for quite a few days and it may seem like your period just won't finish. If you have further symptoms—including increased pain, feel faint or dizzy, or experience discomfort in one shoulder—you should contact your doctor immediately. Even though the embryo is not in the uterus it continues to grow, and there is a danger that it can rupture the fallopian tube and cause internal bleeding which, if untreated, can be life-threatening. Where this happens immediate surgery is required.

In the majority of cases, however, your ectopic pregnancy will be identified before there is any danger of a rupture, and you will be admitted to hospital pretty soon after it is diagnosed to have it removed. This is usually done by laparoscopy under a general anaesthetic and, in many cases, the tube is also removed. You will normally be in and out of the hospital in a day, except where you have worse than usual pain or bleeding. Where there is no urgency, and where the pregnancy is very small, it may be possible to treat it with one or more injections of a drug called methotrexate, but this does not always work, and you may end up having surgery anyway.

Doctors do not really have a clear understanding of how an ectopic pregnancy affects future fertility. There is an increased chance of having a second ectopic after you have had the first, because there may be tubal damage. However, most women who have an ectopic pregnancy go on to conceive again and have successful pregnancies. If you do have a tube removed, you have about 75 per cent of the chance you had of conceiving with two tubes (not 50 per cent as is often thought). Emotionally, of course, there is little difference between the experience of an ectopic pregnancy and a miscarriage—the disappointment and the sense of loss are similar (see Chapter 9).

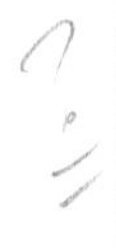

> The infertility specialist said, 'That is your third [miscarriage] so we'd better start some investigations.' He called it 'recurrent miscarriage'—used that language—so suddenly we'd gone from, 'Oh it's an accident and just bad luck', into this really bad space. It was really bloody awful. On the other hand, though, it was a relief, because I did know this wasn't normal, the amount of blood loss, the pain, the tiredness.
>
> Lee

> It took longer to get pregnant the second time, probably five, maybe even seven months. The fear was there in Lee—there was a degree of trepidation about it that wouldn't have been there if it hadn't been for the first miscarriage. Unfortunately, it didn't last terribly long, eight weeks I think, or ten weeks. It fed Lee's conviction there was something amiss. For me it was just a great tragedy. Awful. Lee wanted to keep it secret, she didn't want me to tell anybody, perhaps about her failure, perhaps it was too personal, and she had to deal with it first.
>
> Mark

> It's only people who have been there that know miscarriage is common. I only found that out through my experience. I didn't think it was that unlikely to happen, but I had no idea it was so common, or that you need three before the medical people start questioning it.
>
> Mark

Recurrent miscarriage

Sometimes a single or repeated miscarriage can turn into a series of miscarriages—doctors define *recurrent miscarriage* as at least three in a row, with no successful pregnancy in between. This is fairly rare, however, only affecting fewer than 1 per cent of women. Most of these women will eventually have a successful pregnancy if they keep trying—as long as they are not too old.

Where recurrent miscarriage happens, most doctors will run tests to see whether they can identify a specific cause. In less than 50 per cent of cases they may be able to isolate the cause and—depending on what it is—provide treatment to help maintain the pregnancy next time. In some cases, they may identify a problem that will make it harder than usual to conceive, but it is very rare for that problem to be insurmountable. In the other 50 per cent of cases they may not be able to identify any cause.

All miscarriage is difficult to deal with, but recurrent miscarriage is especially tough. You may feel you've only just got over the last one—whether it was two months or two years ago—and now you are thrown back into all that sadness and grief; the huge disappointment, the feelings of failure, the erosion of self-esteem, the sense of despair. On top of all that, you have to cope with the physical effects of the miscarriage: the bleeding, the cramps and pain, the fatigue, the overnight stay in hospital and the aftermath of all that.

For many people, though, the most difficult thing about recurrent miscarriage is the fact that it knocks a hole in your confidence; it makes you start to lose hope. Where you could put one miscarriage down to bad luck, a second or third inevitably leaves you wondering whether you'll ever be able to carry a baby to term. Your doctor might well say there is no cause for concern yet, but this won't always stop you worrying.

In the end, the limiting factor as to whether you end up with a baby is likely to be how long you are willing to keep trying, and how many miscarriages you can go through. Certainly, women have had babies after having six, eight or even ten miscarriages, though clearly that is not a realistic option for most people. Recurrent miscarriage takes an enormous physical and emotional toll, and there is a limit for everyone. Most women who experience recurrent miscarriage, however, still end up with a baby—either because treatment helps, or just because they keep trying and, for reasons that no one can really explain, on one occasion it works.

One of the frustrations of recurrent pregnancy loss is that, because miscarriages occur so frequently, your doctor is unlikely to do any investigations until you've had at least two or three. If, at this point, your doctor finds an identifiable, treatable cause, you will feel like you have gone through all the pain and grief of those miscarriages unnecessarily. The problem is, of course, that you don't know this until after the fact. If you found the experience of miscarriage particularly tough, or you have reason to suspect something might be wrong, or if you are older, you might talk to your doctor about starting investigations earlier—say after two, rather than three, miscarriages.

Miscarriage—like infertility generally—is one of those things that most people who have never experienced it don't really understand. You may find friends and family have no idea about what you are really going through, and you will inevitably have to deal with those well-meant, but unhelpful platitudes, 'better luck next time', and 'it wasn't meant to be'. It's important to talk to each other at this time, or to a counsellor, a close friend, and/or a support group. There are also a lot of books out there that deal specifically with miscarriage, and these may help.

Causes of recurrent loss

The causes of recurrent miscarriage are complex. There are certain things that doctors know and can identify and treat; there are other things they still don't fully understand. Broadly, the known causes are anatomical, chromosomal, hormonal and related to immune disorders. There are a number of investigations your doctor can do to see whether any of these apply in your case. A blood test is used to diagnose auto-immune disorders, and a hysteroscopy (see Chapter 1) can identify any anatomical problems that may be interfering with pregnancy. If your doctor suspects there may be a chromosomal problem, they will suggest running a *karyotype* analysis of both partners, or of the miscarriage tissue (see below).

Chromosomal abnormalities

The most common type of miscarriage—about 50 per cent of cases—result from random chromosomal error known as *aneuploidy*. To produce a healthy embryo, the egg and sperm must each carry 23 chromosomes which come together to make 23 pairs, or 46 chromosomes, which form the basis of our genetic make-up. Aneuploidy is where there is an abnormality in the number of chromosomes; one or more of the resulting pairs may have an additional chromosome, *trisomy*, or may have only one chromosome, *monosomy*. In some cases the embryo will survive with the abnormality; for example, where there is an extra 21 chromosome, which will result in Down's Syndrome, or trisomy 21. In most cases where aneuploidy occurs, however, the embryo will not survive and miscarriage will follow. Aneuploidy is a common random occurrence which is not associated with an increased risk of subsequent miscarriage. It can happen to anyone, and it doesn't mean there is something wrong with you.

There is also a less common chromosomal abnormality known as *translocation,* where part of one chromosome is knocked off and ends up attached to another one. The cells in which this occurs can still contain the correct total amount of genetic material and the person in whom it occurs will generally not be aware that translocation has happened. (This is called *balanced translocation*, because the extra bit on one pair is 'balanced' by the missing bit on another.) However, in some cases, when the pairs of chromosomes divide up, the egg or sperm—and hence the embryo—may end up with too much or too little genetic information. This is known as *unbalanced translocation*, and is associated with higher than usual levels of miscarriage. Because this happens once, however, it doesn't necessarily mean that it will happen the next time. In fact, only about 20 per cent of subsequent pregnancies—and very occasionally up to 50 per cent—are likely to be affected in the same way. The condition is relatively rare, affecting 2–4 per cent of people with recurrent miscarriage, and 2 per cent of people with repeated IVF implantation failure.

> I was diagnosed with this antibody thing [antiphospolipid antibodies]. You know, I reckon that's really Freudian that I can't remember the name. I think the notion that there was an antibody in my body, which meant blood didn't get through the placenta to the embryo that was Mark's and my child, and I miscarried . . . that image . . . that this was inside my body . . . that was huge. It was like my own body had betrayed me.
>
> Lee

Auto-immune disorders

Some women test positive for one or more antibodies—known as *antiphospholipid antibodies*—that are associated with an increased

> We got pregnant again, a third time, and that miscarried even earlier, maybe six to eight weeks. In Lee's mind there was something terribly wrong. It turned out to be this antibody that causes blood clots. For Lee it was, how on earth can my body being doing this to me? How can I be let down? What is wrong with me? In spite of all the good, I must be a bad person. She was bitterly, bitterly heartbroken over what this meant, and bitterly disappointed for me, her partner.
>
> Mark

chance of miscarriage. Having these antibodies doesn't mean that you can't successfully carry a baby, just that it might make it more difficult. In normal circumstances, the immune system identifies foreign material, such as viruses and bacteria, and forms antibodies to reject them. Sometimes, however, this system breaks down and healthy cells are rejected by mistake. In women who have antiphospholipid antibodies, the body mistakenly perceives phospholipids—which line the cell membranes, including those on the walls of blood vessel—as foreign substances, and develops antibodies to protect the body from them. It is thought these antibodies cause tiny blood clots to form in the blood vessels of the placenta and, in so doing, block the blood flow through the developing placenta.

The appropriate treatment for antibody disorders is still being researched and debated. Some doctors prescribe a combination of aspirin and heparin, which may cause the blood to thin and reduce the formation of clots. The effectiveness of this treatment is still being tested, and it has certainly not been proven to be beneficial in all cases.

Very rarely—in approximately half a per cent of cases—women suffer from antiphospholipid antibody syndrome, which is different from just having the antibodies present. The syndrome is associated with very high concentrations of antibodies and previous blood clots. Women who suffer from the syndrome will almost definitely be treated with heparin and aspirin, and may experience more considerable difficulties in maintaining a pregnancy.

Anatomical abnormalities

Most minor anatomical problems (endometrial *polyps* and small intrauterine *fibroids*) do not interfere with your capacity to carry a baby. In some circumstances, however—depending on their size and position—they can contribute to miscarriage. A large endometrial polyp, or a large submucus fibroid (see Chapter 3) that protrudes into the uterine cavity, *may* affect implantation and the growth of the foetus. Once the polyp or fibroid is removed, however, you should have every chance of having a successful pregnancy. Anatomical problems of this nature can be detected and treated with hysteroscopy (see Chapter 1).

Extensive *adhesions*, formed as a result of earlier surgery, can also affect your capacity to carry a baby. Whether the problem caused by the adhesions can be overcome will depend on where they occur, and how extensive they are (see Chapter 3). Women who have a *septate* or *bicornuate uterus* (see Chapter 3) may have a slightly higher than usual risk of having a miscarriage. Again, depending on the exact nature of the condition, it may be possible to correct the problem with surgery. Many women who have these conditions do not suffer from recurrent miscarriage, however.

Summing up

- There is a range of circumstances in which a pregnancy may occur but not continue. Spontaneous first trimester miscarriage is relatively common, occurring in approximately 20 per cent of pregnancies irrespective of how those pregnancies are achieved. However, most women who experience early miscarriage go on to conceive again and successfully carry a baby to term.

- Even though miscarriage is relatively common it can, and often does, have a significant emotional impact resulting in feelings of grief and loss. This can be exacerbated if the miscarriage occurs after a couple have spent a long time trying to conceive, or after a cycle of IVF treatment.
- Recurrent miscarriage—usually defined as three or more in a row—can be even more difficult and can have an enormous emotional impact. Doctors generally start investigating whether there may be a particular problem after three miscarriages.
- Causes of recurrent miscarriage may be anatomical, chromosomal, hormonal or result from antibody disorders. Where a specific cause is identified, treatment may be available, depending on the particular circumstances.

6

Trying again

Further treatment options

About 20 per cent of people who undergo IVF treatment conceive the first time—the rest don't. This figure may be more or less depending on your age. Many more people, however, will conceive as a result of doing repeated cycles; approximately 45 per cent of those people undergoing IVF will be pregnant after four cycles. Your chances of conceiving don't start to go down until you've had around 10 to 15 embryos transferred—between five to eight cycles of treatment. In most cases, the best chance you have of getting pregnant is to repeat your treatment. There are still many things doctors don't know about how all this works, and many factors are beyond their control. Sometimes, you just have to let things run a while.

At some stage after a negative pregnancy test you should arrange to see your specialist to review your previous cycle and plan your next round of treatment. There may be things that your doctor discovered as a result of the first cycle that can help in deciding the best way to proceed from here. They may even have identified a particular problem, and suggest you or your partner undergo some other surgical or medical treatment before you try another cycle. Now that you've done a cycle you will begin to have a better understanding of how everything works, so you can start to participate more actively in decisions about your treatment.

If you have had any form of stimulated cycle, you will probably have to take a month or two off, to give your body a chance to recover and for your menstrual cycle to return to normal. If you have had a natural cycle you can normally begin another round of treatment the following month. If you have frozen embryos from your last cycle, your doctor will usually recommend doing a natural or artificial thaw cycle (see below). If not, they may well suggest repeating the first treatment cycle, or repeating it with some variation, though usually your doctor will only change things after a few repeated cycles. They may, for example, prescribe a higher dosage of the stimulation drugs if you didn't produce many mature eggs the first time, or a lower dosage if you suffered from any degree of *ovarian hyperstimulation syndrome* (OHSS). They may want to try a different *protocol*—perhaps a natural rather than a stimulated cycle. They may suggest fertilising your eggs using *intracytoplasmic sperm injection* (ICSI), rather than allowing them to fertilise naturally. They may suggest transferring two embryos if only one was transferred the first time. They may suggest changing how they do your transfer if there was a problem with that, or they may increase the dosage or type of your luteal support.

Repeating IVF cycles

All IVF treatment cycles are demanding, but for many people the real challenges start to kick in with repeated cycles. The initial enthusiasm and optimism wears off and the reality of daily injections, regular visits to the clinic, the side effects of the drugs and the enormous financial costs, takes over. In some ways, knowing what to expect can make things easier—at least you feel a bit more prepared this time—but it might also make things more difficult—another round of those awful jabs, those hot flushes and headaches. It can also be frustrating not knowing why it isn't working—after all those tests and investigations you'd think they might know.

Pretty much everybody finds undergoing repeated cycles of IVF treatment emotionally and physically draining. This is the time to call on your support networks, to start talking to other people if you haven't already, to slow down the pace of your life, to focus on each other. It's the time to take care of your relationship, to talk openly and honestly, to think about your respective coping mechanisms (see Chapter 9). However you are coping, it might also be a good time to see a clinic counsellor.

> I found the emotional side incredibly hard to deal with—far more than the physical. After the first four failed cycles, I was just devastated every time it didn't work, just really devastated. It was like a roller-coaster. I started off very optimistic, but the first cycle didn't work—I was fine about that. The second time—I remember I was fine about that. Third time . . . I'd always get excited when I did a new cycle because we were always trying something different, but after the third cycle I started to panic. I was getting the numbers, I mean I was getting lots of eggs, they were fertilising, they were growing to blastocysts and I still wasn't getting pregnant, so I thought, 'Something's wrong—there's something not right'.
>
> Andrea

Natural thaw cycle

If you have done an earlier stimulated cycle you may have produced extra embryos that were frozen to be used next time.

It was getting too much. We just said this is all starting to get way too hard. We know that at some point this won't be an option any more, but we just needed a break because we'd been in and out of bloody hospitals from when I was first diagnosed [with testicular cancer] right through to the end of cycle six. If it wasn't the Peter MacCallum Institute, it was Monash. In one week, I remember, we'd spent five days out of seven at one hospital or the other. We just thought, this is bullshit, this is not how people live—people do not live like this. We need to take a break.

Andrew

We chipped away, doing all these different things, but it still wasn't working. There was no reason. The worst part was we'd done all these extra things and we were no further forward in terms of our expectations than we were at the outset. Then when you get to number six and it's still not happening, suddenly statistics start to play a big role and we've moved to the point where we should be pregnant by now. We have no explanation. No one can tell you why it's not happening. That's the worse part. Virtually for everything else in medical science you can get a reason, but not conception. It just didn't happen. That's why it's called the 'miracle of life'.

Andrew

With a *natural thaw* (or 'frozen') *cycle* you do not have to undergo any of the suppression or stimulation—so no nasal sprays or injections—as you already have your embryos. This means a less invasive, shorter and much less expensive cycle. Not all stimulated cycles will produce extra embryos, however, and not all extra embryos will survive the thawing process. Thawing rates vary, but

We didn't muck around with any of the other protocols because we had limited amounts of sperm, so we were already starting fairly high up the scale in terms of the technology. I was always saying, 'Now, what more can we do?' There always was something and, in the end, we did the hamburger with the lot and that's what worked.

Andrew

It was our first cycle so I didn't really know what the numbers [of eggs and fertilised embryos] meant, but apparently it was pretty good. We had 11 embryos. Two were transferred and nine frozen. It was all pretty exciting and then Tracy comes out of the toilet crying and I know what's going on and that was pretty depressing. And then, you know, oh well, we'll try again. Which we did.

Greg

After one particular failed thaw cycle I didn't want to wait a month before trying again. I think I was just a bit obsessed at the time. I just wanted to do it again. I rang the clinic and they said, 'No. You have to wait.' I was doing frozen cycles, so there was no stimulation. I rang again and insisted that I be allowed and they got back to me and said, okay. I don't think I had become more assertive, I think maybe it was a state of emotional frenzy! I think as I went along I learnt more about what questions to ask.

Tracy

you can normally expect about 60 per cent of your embryos to survive.

In a natural thaw cycle the clinic will try to work out when you ovulate based on the length of your cycle. It is helpful to keep a record of the dates of your previous cycles in order to do this. Most

> We did a talk at Monash to other couples doing IVF and on that particular night we followed on from an IVF specialist who said if you haven't got there by cycle six, forget it. He walks out of the room and the first thing we say is that we got pregnant on cycle number seven, so follow what you need to do. Follow your own path, because if we'd paid attention to that this little lad wouldn't be here.
>
> Andrew

> My advice generally would always be to get a second opinion. You don't owe any loyalty to your doctor. Do not roll over and play dead. Be enquiring. Ask questions. Don't just take whatever they give you. Sometimes you might want to push them a little bit to say, 'Well look, is there anything else that we can do?'
>
> Andrea

people start by tracking their ovulation with a urine testing kit. You then have a scan or blood test two to three days before your natural LH surge is expected to check your follicle development and the lining of your uterus. One or more blood tests may also be required to monitor your hormone levels.

The exact timing of your treatment will depend on your follicle size and on the lining of the uterus. You will normally have your transfer two to three days after your LH surge has been detected, depending on the stage of your embryos. If you have a day 2 embryo it must be transferred two days after ovulation, if you have a day 3 embryo, it must be transferred three days afterwards. Your embryos will be thawed—one at a time—either on the day before your transfer or on the morning of your transfer—and maintained under controlled conditions until the transfer. Occasionally, your embryos won't survive and your transfer will have to be cancelled.

Artificial thaw cycle

If your menstrual cycle is irregular, or if you live a long way from your clinic, or if you want to manage the timing of your treatment for a particular reason, your doctor may suggest an *artificial thaw cycle*. An artificial thaw mimics the body's natural cycle and uses drugs to fool the body into thinking it is producing a follicle and ovulating. You begin by taking oestrogen tablets on day 3 to 5 of your cycle for about ten to 12 days to thicken the lining of your uterus. Normally, a developing follicle secretes oestrogen to do this job. You then have a scan to check the lining is thickening adequately and that there is no follicle development.

You then start using progesterone pessaries which, because you normally produce progesterone at ovulation, lets the body think it has ovulated. The transfer is done two to three days after the start of pessaries, which allows for some control and flexibility. You continue the oestrogen and progesterone until you have a pregnancy test. Because of the progesterone, you will not normally have a bleed or period, which means you must have a blood test to determine pregnancy. If you do get a bleed or period, or have any spotting, you should call your clinic.

If the test is positive and you are pregnant, you continue with both drugs until you are between eight to 12 weeks pregnant. If the test is negative you will normally stop straightaway, but make sure you confirm this with your clinic before you do. Once you have stopped the pessaries, you will have a bleed approximately two to four days later.

Additional treatment

There are some additional tests and techniques available that your doctor may recommend at some point in your treatment depending on your particular circumstances. These include a *hysteroscopy* or *laparoscopy* (see Chapter 1)—if you haven't already had one—blastocyst transfer, assisted hatching, karyotype testing and pre-implantation genetic diagnosis (PGD). A doctor may suggest new or different treatment protocols that are considered 'experimental' or 'cutting edge.' If this is the case, it is important to get a second or third opinion from a different specialist, perhaps even from a different clinic.

Blastocyst transfers

Blastocyst is the name given to the large group of cells—over one hundred—that form the embryo approximately five days after fertilisation of the egg by the sperm. This is the stage immediately before an embryo implants into the wall of the uterus. For many years scientists could only maintain an embryo outside the body for two or three days—to about the eight-cell stage. This is the time when most clinics used to transfer the embryo to the woman. In recent years, improvements to the culture medium in which embryos are nurtured have enabled scientists to grow the embryo to this more advanced stage in vitro.

Increasingly, many clinics recommend having blastocyst transfers fairly early in the course of your treatment, though some still do a few standard day two or three transfers before recommending it. The aim of blastocyst transfers is to enable scientists to monitor the development of the embryos for longer, so they can more accurately assess which embryos are the most healthy. The process doesn't produce better embryos, but it allows the scientist to identify and screen out those embryos that don't look like they are going to develop further. However, because the embryos spend longer in the culture medium, there is a higher chance of losing some or all of them before they are either transferred or frozen. There is a risk, in fact, that none of the embryos will actually develop to blastocyst stage. Where this happens, you will have gone through a whole treatment cycle and ended up not having a transfer, and not having any embryos to freeze for the next cycle. If your embryos survive the longer time in culture and do reach blastocyst stage, however, you may have an increased chance of getting pregnant, though the evidence for this is not yet conclusive. Some research suggests, in fact, that day 2 or 3 transfers are still more successful than blastocysts. You need to make an assessment, in consultation with your doctor, about the level of risk and chances of success in your particular circumstances.

Assisted hatching

Assisted hatching is a technique that some doctors may suggest when you have had a number of unsuccessful embryo transfers, or where the woman is older or known to have a thicker than usual *zona pellucida* (the outer shell of the embryo). Assisted hatching involves making an opening in the zona pellucida with the aim of giving the embryo a better chance of emerging—or hatching—and implanting into the uterus. There are different techniques for creating the opening, including using a needle, a laser or a chemical solution. Assisted hatching is generally performed on day 3 after fertilisation, when the embryo is at least six cells. It can be performed on both fresh or frozen embryos, and is normally done one to two hours before transfer. The evidence as to whether assisted hatching actually results in increased pregnancy rates, however, is inconclusive, and you may find it is recommended less frequently in the future.

Karyotype testing

A *karyotype* is a systematised diagram of chromosomes. A karyotype test involves taking a sample of tissue cells, placing it in a culture medium and allowing the cells to multiply. After a time, the chromosomes of those cells can be seen under a microscope and examined for abnormalities. Your doctor may suggest doing a karyotype analysis after three miscarriages or a number of unsuccessful IVF embryo transfers.

A karyotype of both partners will identify any underlying chromosomal abnormalities. In about 2–3 per cent of cases, either you or your partner may have an abnormality that would not in other circumstances have any affect on you (ordinarily you wouldn't even know about it) but it affects your capacity to conceive and carry a healthy child. If a problem is identified, your doctor may recommend using pre-implantation genetic diagnosis (see below) which can overcome some chromosomal problems, but not all of them, and should enable you to identify which embryos are the healthy ones. If the problem is more significant, your doctor may suggest you think about using donor eggs or donor sperm.

Alternatively, where there is recurrent miscarriage, your doctor might suggest karyotyping some tissue from the miscarriage. This can identify chromosomal abnormalities in the foetus itself, and may help to explain why the miscarriage occurred. However, it usually indicates a random problem—in which case there's not much that can be done—but occasionally it identifies an underlying ongoing problem.

Pre-implantation genetic diagnosis

Pre-implantation genetic diagnosis (PGD)—sometimes called pre-embryo microbiopsy—may be recommended for couples who are at risk of passing on a genetic abnormality to their child, or for couples who have experienced repeated implantation failure, or where the woman is of advanced age. As with blastocyst transfers, PGD would only normally be recommended if you are producing a reasonable number of eggs. It is used in conjunction with a stimulated IVF cycle.

Your eggs are picked-up in the usual way, fertilised and placed in a culture medium. On day 3 after fertilisation (when the embryos are at least six to eight cells) one cell is removed from each embryo. The removal of a single cell should not cause any damage to the embryo which, if healthy, should continue to develop as normal.

A normal pattern of chromosomes is 23 pairs, one of which determines sex: 46XX for a woman and 46XY for a man. One of the uses of PGD is to identify *aneuploidy.* Aneuploidy is where there is a problem with the number of these chromosomes. If there are more or less than this expected number, abnormalities will occur. PGD can also identify the sex of an embryo so that sex-linked diseases can be screened out, and can identify problems associated with single genes. Haemophilia, Duchenne muscular dystrophy, Tay Sachs disease, cystic fibrosis and thalassaemia can all be identified using PGD.

Apart from screening out specific diseases, PGD enables your doctor to ensure that only chromosomally healthy embryos are transferred, which may reduce your chances of repeated implantation failure. Increasingly, a new and more thorough test using PGD, known as *comparative genome hybridisation* (CGH) is being used and may be an option for more couples in the future. This test can detect abnormalities in all 23 of the chromosome pairs, while other techniques can only detect problems with a few chromosomes.

Donor sperm, eggs and embryos

There is a range of circumstances in which you might consider using sperm, eggs or embryos that have been provided by a donor. In some cases you might know very early on in your attempts to start a family that your best or only chance of conceiving involves using a donor: if you have been identified as having no eggs or no sperm, if there is a significant problem with either your eggs or sperm, or if there is a risk of passing on a genetic disease. In other cases, using donor *gametes* or embryos may not present itself as an option until much later, when you have tried other treatments over a period of time which have not been successful.

Whatever your circumstances, using sperm, eggs or embryos provided by someone else raises all sorts of complex emotional and personal issues. It can come as quite a shock to realise that, while you still may be able to have a family, you won't create your family in the way you always imagined; your children won't be genetically related to one or both of you. You will inevitably feel a sense of loss that your child won't be part of the both of you, that he or she won't have a genetic link to one or both sides of your family, that they won't look like or share certain attributes with either you or your partner. It's not uncommon to feel that even though donor gametes might enable you to have a family, that's not quite the same as having children related to you both, conceived in the same way as everybody else. It's not uncommon for people for whom the only option of having a family is to use donor gametes to feel a bit cheated.

It's also not uncommon for one partner to feel differently from the other about the prospect of using donor gametes. A woman might embrace the idea of using donor sperm quite quickly, while her husband or partner may need more time to work through the implications for him. Or she may need time to adjust to the idea of using sperm from a man with whom she has no relationship—lots of women struggle with the idea of having sperm inside them that is not their partner's. Similarly, a man might be happy to use donor eggs, while his wife or partner will need time to work through the implications for her, or he may struggle with the notion of his child having no genetic link with his partner, or to the idea of his sperm fertilising another woman's egg. Don't be surprised if, at first, you don't see things the same way; you'll both need a bit of time and space to work through all these issues.

Some couples will choose not to go down this path for all sorts of reasons. They might not want to put themselves through assisted conception or IVF, or they might feel the biological link between parent and child is just too important, or they might be happy to pursue other life plans together. For others, though, trying to conceive using donor gametes is a positive step forward in their attempts to create a family. They may feel the genetic link is less important and that using a donor is a way of fulfilling a long-held dream. They might feel they will love and delight in this child irrespective of its biological origins. Many couples have successfully—and very happily—used donor gametes or embryos to create their families.

If you are considering using donor gametes or donor embryos, you will be required to see a counsellor at your clinic. The issues involved are huge—identity, heredity, self-esteem, your role in your relationship and, maybe, even your role in life. The counsellor should guide you through the personal and emotional implications of using a donor, as well as explaining the practical and legal aspects of how it all works. Their job is to make sure you are provided with all the information you need, and that you have the opportunity to talk things through, so you can be confident of making informed decisions about what's best for you and your child.

The issues raised are not likely to be resolved with one conversation and it's important to allow yourselves all the time you need to deal with them thoroughly. If you don't, you risk problems arising if and when you do conceive, or when a baby is born, problems that might have been easier to deal with earlier on. Many people find that a lot of discussion happens after they have left the counsellor's office: in the car on the way home or over dinner that evening. You might also find you need time and space to mull things over on your own, or to talk to other people, before talking to each other again.

If you are considering using donor gametes or embryos after a long period of infertility treatment, you might find dealing with these issues even more difficult. More than likely, by the time you get to this stage you will be pretty exhausted, physically and emotionally. You might not be very keen on the idea of having to go through even more counselling, or of talking through a whole new batch of 'issues'. You may be feeling the pressure of time, and you may feel that sitting around *talking* about your options is the last thing you want to do. While you might be willing to give donor gametes a try, after all this time your expectations might not be very high. For all these reasons, it may be difficult for you to take the necessary time to work through all the implications of using a donor, to think about what it really means for you to parent a child with whom you are not biologically related. You need to balance the race against your biological clock with the necessity of ensuring both partners have explored all the issues and are wholly comfortable with the decision to proceed using a donor.

> They said I would definitely need an egg donor. I had no chance of conceiving myself because I wasn't producing any eggs. At that time I think I was very matter of fact about it. My sister-in-law offered straightaway, so that probably counteracted any major feelings. I suppose there wasn't enough time for me to go through that 'I'm not going to be able to have a child', because I thought, 'Oh well she's donating, it's all going to work'.
>
> Tanya

> I remember one night we talked about maybe using anonymous donor sperm and I thought at first, 'I don't have a problem with that', but then I had to work through it all in my head, you know, the whole thing about carrying a child that you don't know the father of. The concept was fine, but the reality took a bit of getting used to.
>
> Hannah

Known, anonymous and identity-release donors

A donor may be known, anonymous, or identity-release. A known donor is someone personally known to you—a friend or family member—who agrees to provide eggs or sperm in order to help you conceive. A known donor would normally go along to the clinic with you and would have to participate in counselling and undergo a full medical screening process.

An anonymous donor is someone who agrees to provide sperm to a clinic, and about whom you are provided with certain non-identifying details. You are normally told their physical characteristics, medical history and, in some instances, additional personal information, including why they have chosen to donate. With an anonymous donor you cannot find out who they are, or any information that might help you to identify them. In some cases, you may be able to access identifying information if the donor consents, but your child does not have an automatic right to that information. Some clinics using anonymous donors have established voluntary registers where donors agree that information can be released to their biological child when he or she is 18, or earlier if all the parties agree.

An identity-release donor is someone who agrees to provide sperm to a clinic, and about whom you are provided with the same non-identifying information as an anonymous donor. However, when the child is 18 (or earlier by the consent of all the parties), the child has the right to find out the identity of the donor. This may be done either through a formal process of central registration—as is currently done in Victoria—or through the individual clinics. In Victoria, identifying details about all donors who donate to a clinic are placed on a central register. When the child reaches 18 he or she can legally access that information; no further consent is required from the donor and the donor cannot stop that information being released. The donor cannot access identifying information about the donor recipient or the child without their consent. If the donor and the donor recipient agree, that information can be released before the child is 18. Given the generally perceived importance of being able to access this information, for adolescents particularly, there are moves to reduce the age at which the child can access the information.

In all other states and territories, individual clinics manage the storing and release of information. There is a shift, however, towards the Victorian model, with some states (including New South Wales) already in the process of moving towards identity-release for all donors. The current trend in thinking is that it is extremely important for children born of donor gametes to have access to information about their biological origins (see 'What and when to tell your child', below). You need to check with your clinic to find out exactly what information you can access and when.

Where a donor gamete is provided to a couple either through a personal connection or through a clinic—irrespective of whether the donor is anonymous or identity-release—there is no legal relationship between the donor and any child born from that gamete. The donor signs legal consent forms to the use of their gametes and gives up all legal rights to any child born from them. Any child born from the donated gamete legally belongs to the recipient couple.

> If I was successful I wanted my child to know that Lynda [sister-in-law] was the person who had donated, that she had given something of herself. That was important to me. We discussed at what age we would tell the child. She had a little boy who was about one year old at that stage and we decided they would know there was a direct link between them.
>
> Tanya

When and what to tell your child

There is no right or wrong way to tell your child about their conception and each family will decide what's best for them. *What* you tell your child may be influenced by your own level of confidence in your decision to use a donor, on who else among your family and friends knows, and on what access you have to information about the donor. *When* you tell them will depend on your child's level of maturity, their understanding of how families are created, and on questions they may ask. Parents do find the right time and the appropriate words.

There is emerging research to suggest that it is best to tell children early. Young children tend to incorporate the information into their lives much more easily. They learn that families are created in all sorts of ways and theirs is made in this particular way. It is no big deal and becomes something they will have always 'just known'. The research suggests that this is preferable to telling them as they enter adolescence and start dealing with their own issues of identity. Often, just knowing they *could* contact their biological parent can be enormously helpful, whether they actually choose to make contact or not. It is also important for some people to have access to information about their potential for carrying genetic diseases and other inheritable conditions. (There is an illustrated book explaining egg donor conception to young children, *Sometimes it Takes Three*, written by Kate Bourne and published by Melbourne IVF.)

Donor sperm

Donor sperm may be used if:

- the man does not produce any sperm
- there is a risk of passing on a genetic condition
- there are other male factor fertility problems resulting from chemotherapy or other treatment, illnesses or surgery
- there have been a number of repeated cycles of treatment with IVF and ICSI without success
- a man is HIV positive.

Using donor sperm means that any child you conceive will have only the mother's genetic material and not the father's. It is not uncommon for men faced with the possibility of using donor sperm to experience a whole range of feelings, including a sense of inadequacy, low self-esteem, diminished masculinity, grief, loss, frustration and anger. Fathering children is still very much tied up with what it means to be a man, and for many men facing the fact that this is not going to happen for them can be very difficult (see Chapter 9). With time and support, however, many of these issues can be worked through. After some initial doubts and concerns many men are happy to proceed using donor sperm.

> It was during this time that we started to think about using donor sperm. Two of my brothers and their families were coming to Australia for a holiday, so we thought instead of anonymous sperm, it would obviously be better to keep it in the family, to use someone we know. Hannah was much more comfortable knowing the person and I didn't have a problem with it. I have three older brothers, so I rang one and right off he said, 'Yeah, no problem,' and I said, 'No, you have to talk to Jane (who is his wife), you're going to have to talk it over with her.' Hannah and I got them thinking about the implications, you know, how he would regard the baby and would he have any expectations? Then I rang my other brother and he said right away, 'Yeah,' and the same thing . . . I said, 'You'll have to talk to Danielle.' Then I rang my third brother and said, 'Look, I'm not asking you because you're not coming for a visit, but I didn't want you to feel left out!'
>
> Charles

> I guess I'm surprised at the number of people who don't even consider using a brother-in-law as a donor. I've not really heard of many people doing that.
>
> Hannah

Using a known sperm donor

Some couples prefer the idea of using sperm from a known donor, rather than from an anonymous donor. Most often they ask a brother

> We didn't want to pressure anyone [into sperm donation] but once we started talking about it, I think my sisters-in-law felt much closer to us, which was really nice. They became much more involved and it really hit them what we'd been going through.
>
> Hannah

> My brother thought, 'It's just sperm', and I think you either have that clear definition of 'not mine' or you don't.
>
> Charles

or brother-in-law of the male partner, or sometimes they may ask the father. This way a genetic link may be maintained or, at least, the couple feel they are 'keeping it in the family'. Many couples like the idea that there will be an ongoing relationship between the donor and the child.

Asking someone to be a donor, however, is a big step, and agreeing to be one is even bigger; it represents a shift in the nature of the relationship between the woman and her brother-in-law or friend, and it will take time and sensitivity to work through all the questions that will inevitably come up. If you are going to use a known sperm donor, there are some specific things you need to think about in addition to the general issues involved: whom among family and friends you are going tell, what you plan to tell your child and when, and what you expect the relationship between the donor and the child to be.

If your donor agrees to provide sperm he will be required to see a counsellor to make sure he is aware of the various personal and legal implications. If he has a partner or is married, she must also see a counsellor and agree to the donation; and both of them must sign legal consent forms. The donor is required to have a medical consultation and will be screened for any genetic or infectious diseases. He will be required to provide a sperm sample which will be analysed (see Chapter 1). If he is accepted, his sperm will be frozen and quarantined for six months and he will be tested again at the end of that period. If all the tests are still negative, the sperm will be released to the couple. It will remain frozen in storage until it is needed to fertilise the eggs. The donor, or his wife, can change their minds and withdraw their consent at any time up to the time that the sperm is used to fertilise the egg.

Anonymous or identity-release sperm donors

Some couples do not have access to a known sperm donor, or prefer to use an anonymous or identity-release sperm donor. Sperm is available in Australia at the moment though it is not plentiful and you may not have a wide choice; many clinics have an ongoing problem maintaining a reasonable supply. Most couples want to match the physical characteristics of the donor with those of the husband or partner, but this will depend on the number and type of donors available at any given time. Your clinic should provide a range of information about the donors it has available, including their physical characteristics—height, weight, build, skin, hair and eye colour—and may also include some additional personal information.

Issues raised by using a sperm donor

Whether you are planning to use a known, anonymous or identity-release sperm donor there are a number of issues you need to address. The following questions should form the basis of your discussion, both with the counsellor and among yourselves.

- If using donor sperm is your only option, how have you both coped with your diagnosis of infertility and what impact has that had on your relationship?

- If you have been having treatment, how are you both coping generally?
- Have you experienced repeated loss and disappointment and what effect has that had on you both?
- How much energy do you have left to explore this possibility?
- Do you both agree this is your best option?
- Is either partner feeling pressured in any way?
- How do you feel about giving up the chance of conceiving with your own/your partner's sperm?
- What are the emotional implications for both of you of conceiving a child who will not be the biological offspring of its father?
- Who among your family and friends are you going to tell?
- How and when will you tell them?
- How do you think they'll react, and how will you deal with their reactions?
- What will you tell your child in the future, and at what stage might you tell them?
- If the donor is anonymous, what access does your child have to identifying information about him?
- How will you feel if your child wants to find out about their donor in the future, or even meet him?
- If the donor is known, what will the relationship be between the donor and the child?
- What will be the relationship between the child born of the donor sperm, and any other children the donor may have?
- How will this arrangement affect the relationship between the donor and the couple?
- How will other extended family fit in?

The sperm donor procedure

Once you have explored these issues and are ready to proceed, you will normally see your doctor again to confirm your next cycle of treatment, and also meet with the nursing staff to go through the details and day-to-day management of that treatment. Donor sperm can be used for *interuterine insemination* (IUI), or for *gamete intrafallopian transfer* (GIFT) or *in vitro fertilisation* (IVF). Often, to maximise the chances of fertilisation, *intracytoplasmic sperm injection* (ICSI) (see Chapter 4) is used in conjunction with IVF. If you have had previous treatment, you will be familiar with the procedures and the only differences for you will be that, instead of the husband\partner providing the sperm sample, the sperm will already be there, thawing in the lab in time to fertilise your eggs. If your first cycle of treatment is with donor sperm, you need to read Chapter 4 for the details about the type of treatment that has been recommended for you.

> We have been thinking about donor eggs. We want to open up as many options as we can. Instead of just thinking, 'I only want a baby with my partner', I'm thinking of the other options—especially because of the waiting lists. If you do want to use donor eggs, the waiting list is like three years—a ridiculous amount of time—so the quicker you can get over the fact that you're not using your eggs and can get on to the list, the better. But at the same time, you have to feel ready because we started to think about donor eggs and it was all going along fine and I'm like, 'Yeah, yeah I can deal with that'. Then one night I just said to Charles, 'Nah, I'm not ready, I want to do more IVF.' Then I felt guilty because Charles was so willing to give up a biological link to the child and here's me going, 'I want it to be my child.' You've got to be ready.
>
> Hannah

Egg donation

A couple may choose to use donor eggs in a range of circumstances, including:

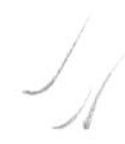

- the woman does not produce any eggs herself
- the eggs she produces are of poor quality
- there is a risk of passing on a serious genetic disease
- there are other female factor fertility problems resulting from chemotherapy or other treatment, illness or surgery
- there have been a number of repeated cycles of treatment without success.

A woman who discovers she has no eggs, or poor quality eggs, may experience similar feelings to those experienced by a man who discovers he has no sperm: a sense of loss and of feeling cheated, a sense of inadequacy and reduced self-esteem, grief, frustration and anger. Even today, motherhood is very closely associated with what it means to be a woman, and it is still commonly regarded as being the ultimate fulfilment for a woman. Acknowledging that you will never have a child to whom you are genetically related, or feeling that your body has let you down, can be difficult and you need to allow yourself time to work through your feelings before you start to think about using donated eggs (see Chapter 9).

Donor eggs may be provided to a couple in a number of different ways. The donor may be known to a couple—often a sister or sister-in-law or close friend; or the donor may be someone who has responded to an advertisement placed by a couple; or the donor may be someone who has donated their eggs to a clinic anonymously and who will not be known to the couple. In Australia at the moment, there are very few anonymous egg donors available and most clinics have a three- to-four-year waiting list. Because of this, couples are increasingly approaching family members or close friends to donate eggs, or advertising (see box). Where a couple provide their own donor, there is no wait for treatment, though the process itself still takes time.

> We had counselling in Melbourne—in all sorts of combinations. There was Lynda [egg donor] and her husband—my brother-in-law—and me and my husband, then my husband and me on our own, and my husband and the donor together, and then all four of us. I think most of our questions came after we left the room. We all went to lunch and discussed it and then had more questions.
>
> Tanya

Advertising for egg donors

Some couples have successfully advertised for an egg donor, and anecdotal evidence suggests the practice may be increasing. If you are considering advertising for a donor, you need to talk to your clinic first to get advice on how to do it safely and legally. In Victoria (but in no other states) advertisements have to be approved by the Ministry of Health and your clinic should explain the process for doing this. They may also suggest ways you can protect yourself, including using a PO Box number for your replies and a mobile phone number, rather than your home phone number. They can also provide advice on the sorts of question you need to ask. Some clinics may act as a go-between for the donor and the couple to keep everything anonymous, and will undertake the initial donor screening. Other clinics may need you to meet the donor yourselves, and present to the clinic together.

Using a known egg donor

Each clinic will have its own policy governing the use of donor eggs, and there are likely to be some variations. Most clinics will make decisions on a case-by-case basis, taking into account the

So we considered anonymous egg donors and we saw the counsellor and went on the waiting list. But then we thought it was stupid to consider an anonymous donor without first asking my sister-in-law, but how do you ask? How do you bring it up? What do you say? So we sort of thought we'd drop in one night and just tell her we were on the waiting list for donor eggs, and say, 'We are not actually asking you, but we don't want you to think we wouldn't consider you if you offered.' We really didn't want to ask but, at the same time, if you don't ask then this anonymous donor comes up and my sister-in-law says 'I would have donated,' you'd be like, 'Oh my God, why didn't we ask?'

Charles

We ended up sitting there for an hour and a half talking [to a potential known egg donor] and her real feelings came out. To a certain extent I think it's such . . . not a privilege, but it's been really nice to go through that, to talk about such personal things with people. It just changes things. It brings you closer. It's been such an interesting time—it's amazing what you can talk to people about and how the relationships can change so much.

Hannah

I have talked with a few people about being possible egg donors and they have been very honest and I am glad. I think that's all you can ask for, and you can't judge people or understand how their mind works. I've always thought, all along, that I don't know if the situation was reversed whether I could donate eggs.

Hannah

individual circumstances of each couple and their donor. The overall process, however, is usually pretty much the same. Clinics generally prefer the donors to have already completed their own families—though this is not always essential—and that the donor is no older than their late thirties. Young donors, in their early twenties, are not normally encouraged. Women who are on the pill or who have had their tubes tied can donate. Donors cannot be paid for their eggs, but all out-of-pocket medical costs are borne by the recipient couple.

Everyone involved in the arrangement—the recipient couple and their donor, and the donor's husband or partner if she has one—has to see a counsellor. The same counsellor will normally see both the recipients and the donor separately in the first instance, and may suggest everyone meets as a group after this initial discussion. This will vary, however, from state to state and clinic to clinic. Both the donor and the couple will need to work through all the legal, personal and emotional issues involved (see below).

All potential egg donors—whether known or anonymous—have to go through a screening process where a counsellor and doctor consider their suitability. Personality and lifestyle factors are normally taken into account, as well as medical and gynaecological history. Counsellors will explore the donor's reasons for donating and—depending on the state you live in—how the donor feels about being contacted by the child when they are eighteen. The potential donor will be informed about the various medical procedures involved and all the legal implications. They will be given the opportunity to raise questions and explore their feelings.

Anonymous or identity-release egg donors

Where a couple does not want to use a known egg donor, or does not have access to a known donor, they may put their names on a waiting list for eggs donated by an anonymous donor. The number of available anonymous egg donors, however, is extremely low and currently does not come close to meeting the needs of infertile couples. Anonymous egg donors have to undergo counselling and extensive, invasive medical procedures for which they cannot legally be paid. It is a time-consuming and complex process that can be

> I'd sort of thought an anonymous egg donor wouldn't be bad, but I'd rather use a known egg donor if I could. But the more we talked about it, the more we thought maybe you are better off with an anonymous donor. I started to think, you know, if you see the known donor all the time—I guess being a woman they do have those maternal instincts—how would they feel towards the child? So I started to think maybe an anonymous donor would be better after all. In a way, being open about it and talking honestly to possible donors brought me around to the other side.
>
> Hannah

difficult to fit into a busy life with work, children and other responsibilities. Because of the long waiting lists, many clinics only offer egg donation to women under a certain age. This cut-off varies, but ranges from about 38 to 45 years of age.

Once you put your name on the list you will generally be asked to contact the clinic periodically—around every three months or so—to confirm that you still want to use donor eggs. Again, this may vary from clinic to clinic. When a donor becomes available you will be notified by the clinic who will provide you with some basic information about the donor. The type of information and the amount of detail will vary, but you should normally expect the same basic physical characteristics that you get with a sperm donor. The clinic will attempt to match physical characteristics to the recipient couple, but this may be difficult with the very limited supply.

As with a known donor, there are many issues that need to be worked through. For the recipient couple, these issues are essentially the same as for using donor sperm (see above) but, as the process for a woman donating eggs is very different from a man donating sperm, there are some additional issues that need to be addressed.

Issues for the egg donor

- Why has she agreed to be a donor?
- Has she come to this decision of her own free will?
- Does she feel under any pressure to be a donor?
- Is there anything in her own history that might influence her decision, a previous termination or miscarriage, for example?
- Is she fully aware of the various medical procedures she will have to undergo, and the possible effects of those procedures?
- How does she feel about the fact that there will be a child in existence that is genetically related to her, but with whom she will have no legal connection?
- If the recipient couple is known, what are her expectations of the relationship between her and the child and between them and her children if she has any?
- Who will be told about the arrangement and what and when will they be told?
- How will this arrangement affect her relationship with the couple?
- How will this arrangement affect relationships with other family members, or close family friends?
- How will she feel if a pregnancy is terminated because of a medical problem or abnormality, or if a child is born with an abnormality, or if no pregnancy results?
- If the donor is anonymous, how does she feel about the possibility the child might contact her in the future?
- What will she tell her family and friends, and her children if she has any?

The egg donor procedure

Once you have worked through these issues and everybody is ready to proceed, you will have to sign consent forms. Your doctor will then arrange the synchronising of your cycle with the donor's cycle.

Whether the donor is anonymous or known, the doctor will see her on her own and run through her medical and gynaecological history. They will check there is no history of inherited genetic disease and arrange testing for Hepatitis B and C and HIV for her and her partner, and other infectious diseases if they feel it is necessary. The recipient couple would also normally undergo testing for these diseases if they haven't already done so.

The donor will then undergo the first part of a stimulated cycle—injections of FSH, blood tests and scans (see Chapter 4)—the aim being to produce as many eggs as is safely possible. At the same time as the donor is being treated, the recipient will also undergo hormone treatment in order to synchronise her cycle with that of the donor. Once synchronised, the donor eggs will be retrieved and fertilised with the husband or partner's sperm. This is usually done by *intra-cytoplamic sperm injection* (ICSI) (see Chapter 4) to maximise the chances of getting as many embryos as possible. On day 2 to 5 after fertilisation, the embryos will be transferred to the recipient's uterus via a catheter. Where synchronising is not possible for some reason, the donor's eggs will be fertilised and the embryos frozen then thawed later and transferred to the recipient at the appropriate time in her cycle. Any embryos that are not transferred can be used for a future cycle.

Once all the embryos are used—or if only very few resulted from the cycle—it may be possible to access further eggs, but this will depend on availability and on your individual circumstances. It would also depend on the willingness of the donor to undergo another cycle of treatment. You would normally have to go back to your doctor and the counsellor to reassess your situation.

Donated embryos

Another option for couples who do not produce eggs, or for whom egg quality is a problem, is to use donated embryos. There is also a long waiting list—though generally not quite as long as for egg donors—and some clinics may place age restrictions on who can go on that list. Donated embryos usually come from couples who have been successful with IVF, have completed their families, and have some remaining embryos in storage. However, the number of embryos available is still very limited.

Couples thinking about using donor embryos need to explore some additional issues. Unlike with sperm or egg donation, there will be no biological link between a child born from a donated embryo and the recipient couple. Also, as many of the couples who donate embryos already have children themselves, any child born to the recipient couple is likely to have full-blood siblings.

These are also issues for the donor couple too who will know that a child, or children, who is genetically theirs, legally belongs to and is being brought up by someone else. They will know their children have a full-blood sibling. If the donor is anonymous, all the same issues about the possibility of a child making contact in the future apply.

The process of using donor embryos—seeing your doctor, talking to a counsellor, going on the list and periodically checking in—is the same as for egg donation. The medical process is actually less complicated, however, because the embryos are already frozen. They need only to be thawed and transferred (see Chapter 4).

Surrogacy

Surrogacy is where a woman carries and gives birth to a baby for another woman who is unable to carry a baby herself. This may be because she has no uterus, or because her uterus is damaged, or because carrying a baby may endanger her life. There are two types of surrogacy. A couple may create an embryo from their own egg and sperm and transfer that embryo to the surrogate mother. In this case there is no genetic link between the surrogate mother and the child born from that embryo. This is sometimes referred to as 'gestational carriage'. In the other instance the surrogate mother provides the egg as well as carrying the baby, so the surrogate does have a genetic link to the baby.

There have been some, though very few, successful cases of surrogacy in Australia. This area is governed by state, rather than federal legislation, so your access to it will depend upon where you live. Currently, it can be undertaken in New South Wales and the Australian Capital Territory, and might possibly be available in some other states, though the legal situation is far from clear. If you feel this is something you want to pursue, you will need to talk to your clinic in the first instance to clarify the legal situation in the state where you live. If it is a possibility, you need to explore it further with one of the counsellors.

Summing up

- Your chances of conceiving increase, the more cycles of treatment you do (up to a point). However, undergoing repeated cycles of treatment over an extended period of time can be emotionally and physically demanding.
- If you have frozen embryos from an earlier cycle you can do a natural or artificial thaw treatment cycle which is less physically demanding because you do not have to go through the stimulation phase, as well as being less expensive.
- There is a range of advanced treatment options from which you may benefit. Increasingly, clinics are using blastocyst transfers where the embryo has been grown on to a more mature stage. Some clinics offer assisted hatching though the evidence for the success of this technique is not conclusive.
- Karyotype testing and pre-implantation genetic diagnosis can be used to determine and overcome certain chromosomal and genetic problems.

- Donor gametes may be used where a couple do not produce their own eggs or sperm, or where there is a significant problem with their eggs or sperm that cannot be overcome by treatment. They may also be used where the cause of infertility is unknown and all other options have been exhausted. Using donor gametes raises a number of significant personal issues that need to be discussed both with each other and with a counsellor.
- Donor gametes may be provided by a person known to the couple, or they may be provided anonymously through an infertility clinic. Laws and regulations regarding what access your child has to identifying information about donors provided through a clinic vary from clinic to clinic and state to state.
- All donors, whether personally known to the couple or provided through a clinic, go through a medical screening process to ensure they and their gametes are healthy. Where the donor is anonymous, basic information about the physical characteristics of the donor is usually provided.
- Using a sperm donor is a relatively straightforward process, while using an egg donor is a lot more difficult and complex. There is currently a long waiting list for egg donors, and increasingly couples are trying to find their own, known egg donors to avoid this lengthy wait.
- It is sometimes possible to use donor embryos, usually provided by couples who have completed their own families and still have embryos left. However, the numbers available are low and waiting lists are long.
- Surrogacy, where a woman carries a baby on behalf of another women, may be possible in some states.

7

Single women and lesbian couples

Options for conceiving

Single women and women in lesbian relationships who want to have a child will obviously approach conception in a rather different way to heterosexual couples. Some single women and lesbians may be able to conceive using a known sperm donor without any intervention from the medical profession. Some may find themselves involved with a doctor or specialist—even though, strictly speaking, they are not 'infertile'—because of a need to access advice and information and/or donor sperm; some may find they have a fertility problem after all—irregularities with ovulation, blocked fallopian tubes or endometriosis do not, of course, discriminate on the basis of marital status or sexuality—and they need medical intervention to help them conceive.

You may be one of the increasing number of single women who are starting to think about having children on your own. Perhaps your focus has been on other things—study, career, travel, life—and only now do you feel you are in a position, emotionally and financially, to have a family. Maybe your biological clock is ticking and, while you don't rule out the possibility of a relationship in the future, there may be only a small window of opportunity for you to conceive. While you may not have imagined having a family on your own, your desire for kids might be strong and this might be your only realistic option.

So, too, are more lesbians having families, either while in a relationship or by themselves. As lesbians are legally considered 'single' for the purpose of access to infertility treatment, your options for conceiving are the same as those for single women.

This chapter explores the options available for conception for single women and lesbians and describes some of the advantages and disadvantages of each. It looks in detail at self insemination with a known donor and outlines the personal, medical and legal issues involved. It explores the implications of using known, anonymous or identity-release donors. It describes what you can expect if you decide to use a specialist infertility clinic, and it explores some of the personal and emotional implications of all this.

The laws and regulations governing who can access services from infertility clinics vary from state to state, and exactly what services are accessible vary from clinic to clinic. There have been numerous changes to these laws in recent years and these changes are ongoing. This chapter provides an overview of the current legal situation, but because of the rapidly changing nature of these laws, it is really important you call clinics directly and clarify exactly what services are available.

The issue of whether single women and lesbians can access medical services to conceive is not un-controversial, and discussions about this have often been accompanied by public debate and media attention.

If you are a single woman—either heterosexual or lesbian—or part of a lesbian couple you cannot get away from the fact that other people will have opinions about your capacity to parent a

> I ended a long-term relationship in my twenties and the next four or five years I found very difficult. Then all of a sudden I was 30. I thought, if I have to go through life without a partner I can do with that, but I will not go through life without children. If I have to cope without being married or without a partner obviously I will—I won't internally combust—but I will if I don't have children.
>
> Wendy

child and, more than likely, will express those opinions at any available opportunity. Sometimes, it can be difficult to ignore this, but it won't be the first time you've had to deal with negative attitudes and you will work out a way of handling it that best suits you. Remember, lots of women have gone before you and, if you need to, there are always people you can turn to for support (see Chapter 10).

If you are single or a lesbian, there are a number of options for trying to conceive. Remember, however, that as the current laws stand, not all these options are available in all states, and you may need to cross borders to access certain services. Your options include:

- sex with a man
- self insemination with a known donor
- insemination at a clinic with your own known donor
- insemination at a clinic with an anonymous or identity-release donor
- insemination at a clinic with low-key medical intervention, low-dose fertility drugs, or assistance with ovulation—with your own known donor, or with an anonymous or identity-release donor
- in vitro fertilisation treatment with your own known donor, or with an anonymous or identity-release donor.

> Some people could not understand why I didn't just go down to the pub and drag someone home and do it that way. There are a multitude of reasons why not. Sure, if I go to the pub three times this week I could bring home three different men, but it's not really what I want to tell my child. I wouldn't want my child to think I'd done that. And I couldn't do it in secret. I couldn't do that to any man. I don't think I have that right. And, apart from anything else, it would be just my luck that I'd contract some terrible disease as well.
>
> Wendy

Sex with a man

Some single women—and some lesbians—may consider having sex with a man to get pregnant with no intention of involving, or even telling, the man concerned—'a one-night stand'. Having unprotected sex with a stranger to get pregnant certainly avoids the need for the complex negotiations required with a known donor, and it is one way of avoiding having to deal with doctors and drugs. For lots of reasons, though, it might not be a great idea.

Conceiving with a stranger means you will know nothing about the personal, family and medical background of the person who will provide half the genetic material for your child. You will have no idea, for example, about their general health, or if there is a family history of inherited disease or psychiatric illness. It is also likely that your child will ask questions about his or her genetic origins later in life, and may also want information about—or even to meet—their biological father. Conception in this way provides no opportunity for this. On a practical note, too, you will not be able to take the usual safe-sex precautions and, therefore, will leave yourself—and your child—vulnerable to sexually transmitted disease, including Hepatitis B and C and HIV. Some women also just do not feel comfortable about intentionally setting out to conceive with a man whom they do not plan to tell should they become pregnant.

Another option may be to have sex with someone you know—perhaps a former partner or an old friend—for the purpose of getting pregnant. In this situation you will, at least, know or have access to information about him and his background and can talk openly about what you want. This sort of arrangement, however, raises the same issues about rights, roles and relationships that apply when you use a known donor (see below). In addition, if you were to conceive with a friend or former partner, he would legally be considered the father of your child.

Using a known donor

A more commonly considered option is using a donor. A donor may be known, anonymous, or identity-release (see Chapter 6). A known donor is someone personally known to you—a friend, colleague or acquaintance—who has agreed to provide sperm in order to help you conceive. The extent to which a known donor has a relationship with the child, or is involved in the child's life is negotiated between you and him and any other relevant parties. It is important to remember, however, that there are legal considerations which may affect any decisions you make. With heterosexual couples any child born of a donor gamete legally belongs to the recipient couple, but this is not the case if you are single or a lesbian. The exact legal relationship between a known donor and your child is, at the moment, subject to some legal debate (see below). It is really important that you get up-to-date legal advice before you use a known donor.

If the donor sperm is provided through a clinic—irrespective of whether he is anonymous or identity-release—there is no legal relationship between the donor and the child. You can legally leave the space on the child's birth certificate for 'father' blank after providing documentation from your clinic. In Western Australia (but nowhere else) it is possible to include both names of a same-sex couple on the birth certificate where the child has been conceived through donor sperm provided by a clinic, though not if the insemination was done privately.

> A lot of children born through donor insemination are going to want to know something about their father. That doesn't mean that the donor will live with you, or parent the child, but having a known donor means that if the child has questions about its genetic origins you can answer them pretty easily.
>
> Kris

> My only non-negotiable thing in all this was that I wanted my child to have access to identifying information about their donor father later in life. I think it's human nature to want to know what your parent looks like. Having an identifiable donor doesn't frighten me. I work with children and I see all sorts of families and I'm not intimidated by what might happen. Whether the child wanted or didn't want contact with the donor, that doesn't frighten me either way. Whatever the child is comfortable with. It's going to be their decision, but I want them to be able to make a decision. I don't want the law to get in their way.
>
> Wendy

Legal status of a known donor

The principal legislation that governs family relationships in Australia is the *Family Law Act 1975* (Cwlth), a federal government

> I wanted a known donor because I wanted my child to know their genetic origin and to have a relationship with their father as well as with their mother. I felt very strongly about that. But how that relationship may unfold, what it might be, I don't know. And that's fine. There will be ongoing discussion and who knows.
>
> Darcy

Act that applies irrespective of the state you live in. The legislation that governs the registration of births differs from state to state. To date, there have been two cases heard in the Family Court which have a bearing on the legal status of known donors. The cases are referred to as *B and J* and *re Patrick*.

B and J involved a lesbian couple who had a baby with a known donor. The name of the known donor was included on the application for a birth certificate and appeared on the actual birth certificate, but the donor and the mothers agreed that he would have no financial or other responsibilities in relation to the child. The birth mother was receiving the single mother's pension, but was informed by the Department of Social Security that payment of her pension would cease unless she applied for child support from the donor. The donor then sought a declaration from the Family Court that he was not a person from whom child support could be sought—that is, he was not a parent. The court held that the donor was not a parent for the purposes of the *Child Support (Assessment) Act 1989* (Cwlth) and could not therefore be required to pay child support.

The decision in this case certainly suggests that a known donor cannot legally be required to provide financial support for a child of whom he is the biological father in a private known donor arrangement. However, it might be wise to treat this decision with some degree of caution; it is only *one* case and *one* judge's opinion. Future case law may enable us to more confidently rely on this decision.

The second case, *re Patrick,* involved a lesbian couple who had had a child using a known donor. After the child was born, the donor applied to the Family Court under the Family Law Act for contact with the child. In this case the judge ruled that, while the known donor was the biological father of the child, he was not a 'parent' for the purpose of the Family Law Act. However, the Family Law Act states that any person concerned with the care, welfare or development of the child can apply to the Family Court for orders in relation to that child. (An order might relate to where the child lives or to contact with the child—what used to be called 'custody' and 'access'.) In *re Patrick*, the court recognised that the donor, though not the legal parent of the child, did have a social and biological relationship with the child and therefore granted him contact over the objections of the child's mothers.

On the basis of this case we can assume that a biological father—irrespective of whether or not his name appears on the birth certificate—can exercise certain rights in relation to his biological child if the court considers that granting those rights is in the best interests of the child. These rights can include regular contact with the child. The bottom line here is that it is reasonable to assume that if a known donor makes an application to the court for some degree of contact with his biological child, the court may well treat such an application favourably and order that contact.

It's always important to remember that the Family Law Act can grant rights to the child that cannot be waived, limited or restricted by any agreement between the donor and the parents. In other words, although you and your donor can and should clearly outline your expectations, and write them down in some form of agreement, the courts will not necessarily enforce that agreement unless they consider it is in the best interests of the child.

Parenting orders

It is possible for any person concerned with the care, welfare or development of a child to apply for a parenting order through the

Family Court. Where a lesbian couple have had a child, the non-biological mother can make an application if she wants to establish some form of legal connection to the child. A parenting order grants certain responsibilities to the applicant in relation to the child which can include residence, contact and decisions about the day-to-day care, welfare and development of the child.

In order to obtain a parenting order you have to see a lawyer, or a court appointed Family and Child Counsellor, and go through a formal process of presenting information and documents to the Family Court. Once the parenting order has been issued, the non-biological mother has certain legal rights and responsibilities that can only be overturned by going back to the Family Court. In practice, this can include the power to authorise medical treatment for the child, sign forms for participation in school trips, enrol the child in day care and take on the numerous other day-to-day parenting responsibilities. Depending on the type of parenting order obtained, this can effectively make the non-biological mother a 'legal guardian' of the child, though this term is no longer used.

Birth certificates

The Registry of Births, Deaths and Marriages in your state or territory is responsible for issuing birth certificates. How each registry deals with an application for a birth certificate that involves a donor varies from state to state—and in practice, may vary with whom you talk to in the office on any given day. This is a relatively new area for the registries and many are still in the process of formulating policy to deal with donor conception.

By law, you must register the birth of a child within 60 days. You are required to fill out a form which asks for information about the date and place of birth, and about the child's mother and father. The registrar then uses the information that you provide to register the birth and complete the birth certificate.

If you have used a known donor in a private arrangement and you include his name on the form where it asks for 'father', his name will appear on the birth certificate. If you write 'known donor' on the registration form, it is uncertain at this stage what additional information you will be asked to provide and what the consequences of this will be. For this reason, you should get local, up-to-date legal advice before you register the birth.

If you have used an anonymous donor through a clinic—whether identity release or not—you can write 'anonymous donor' on the application form. You will then be asked to provide evidence of when and where you received treatment—this can normally be dealt with by a letter from your clinic. In this case, 'anonymous donor' will not appear on the birth certificate—the 'father' box will simply be left blank. In some cases it may be possible to get the non-biological mother's name on the birth certificate, not as an additional 'mother' or 'parent', but in section six of the birth certificate which is entitled Informant. For example, in Victoria, if details of the non-biological mother are included on the application form and she signs it, her name and address may be included in this section of the birth certificate. In Western Australia if a baby is conceived through a clinic both mothers' names can be listed on the certificate.

It is important to remember that it is an offence to knowingly submit incorrect or false information on the application form. This means that if you know who the biological father of your child is, it is an offence to state 'unknown'—or anything similar—on the form. If you do state that the father is 'unknown', you will almost certainly be asked to explain why you do not know his identity.

Self insemination with a known donor

Irrespective of the complex legal issues, many single women and many lesbians—whether single or in a relationship—start by looking for a known donor. This method has the advantages of being private, cheap and non-invasive. You can do it at home and have complete control over all aspects of the procedure, including how it is done and who else knows. If it works, it can be a quick and convenient solution, and it certainly avoids having to deal with infertility clinics and counsellors.

While all this might be true, however, finding and negotiating with a known donor is not as easy, or as uncomplicated, as it might first appear. There is a range of medical, legal and personal issues that need to be explored long before conception is attempted.

> I looked at the ads in the gay press and contacted a man from there. We met and, in fact, came very close to trying, but in the end I asked myself, 'Can I have this man in my life? Would I be comfortable with that?' And I decided that I wouldn't be, so I pulled out. There are a lot of dangers in approaching someone through an advertisement. It's a big risk.
>
> Darcy

> Finding a donor was extremely difficult. It was a lengthy process and it took a lot of energy. There were so many things to consider. It is a very risky thing. I do want this person in my life, and in my child's life, so there are a lot of things I had to weigh up.
>
> Darcy

Legal status of self insemination

It is important to note that in Victoria it is illegal for a partner—or in fact anyone other than a doctor or clinician—to do an insemination. It is probably not actually illegal for a woman to do an insemination herself, but this point is still the subject of some legal debate. In Western Australia it is illegal for a person to perform an insemination privately without being under the care of a doctor. In South Australia, it is illegal to perform an insemination without a licence to do so. In all other states and territories there is no legislation that relates to this issue. These regulations may change in the future.

I met with a man, a friend of a friend. First, I had to get to know him. I wanted to feel sure about his role and his intentions and so we talked about him being a donor for quite a while. On a number of occasions we met and had lunch and coffee. We started with, 'Why?' Why does he want to have a child? Why do I want to have a child? What were his intentions? What role did he see himself playing? We talked about frequency of contacts—what he wanted, what I wanted . . . We also talked about the fact that things change, feelings may change . . . The bottom line is being able to talk about all this.

Darcy

There is some fortune and luck in it [choosing a known donor]. I planned as much as I could have planned, but in the end there was still a lot of not knowing.

Darcy

Choosing a known donor

Most people start by looking around their social circle to find a donor—friends, former partners, an older acquaintance who's already had children, or relatives of the non-biological mother. Where there is no one in their social circle, some women have tried advertising for a donor in their local gay press. Anecdotal evidence suggests that this often results in numerous crank or unsavoury phone calls, and is not a particularly good way of finding a suitable donor.

You may want your prospective donor to be of the same racial or ethnic origin as you, or to have particular physical characteristics that go some way to matching yours. You may prefer him to have a similar level of education, or to share the same sort of values and ideas about life. You may want him to come from the same cultural background or even share the same religion. You might want him to be musical, or sporty, or practical or artistic. You may prefer that he is gay or straight. Or, as long as the donor is healthy, none of these things may matter to you at all. You might just want him to be a nice guy, someone you like and respect. You may find—as many women have—that while the physical characteristics of your donor are extremely important at the beginning of this process, the longer you try to conceive, and the more attempts you make, the less important they become.

Many lesbians—and some straight women—choose gay friends to be donors, others might ask straight men with whom they have a current or former relationship. Your prospective donor may be single or part of a couple, he might be older or younger, he may already have fathered children or not. He might live close by or far away, or even overseas. He might be a good friend of both partners, or only really known by one. All these things might influence his decision to provide sperm—and your decision to choose him—and may affect the sorts of arrangements you have if and when a child is born. You will need to take all these factors into account when you make your assessment of whether he is the right person.

Irrespective of any of this, two things are of paramount importance: the medical health of your donor and his sperm—both now and in the past—and the level of openness, trust, respect and communication you share. These should be the most important considerations in making your choice. Once you start talking to any prospective donor, you will find all sorts of things crop up that you hadn't even thought about. Being able to openly and honestly discuss what can be highly personal, intimate or challenging issues is essential. You will need to have full, frank and frequent discussions with everyone involved, and without a good level of trust and friendship, this will be very difficult.

Asking someone to be a sperm donor—and agreeing to be one—is a big deal, irrespective of whether you anticipate your donor having a very limited or a very significant involvement with your child. Although it might not seem so at first, there are some huge issues you're going to have to deal with. Conceiving with a sperm donor might not be the traditional way of making a baby, but it still involves the participation of two people; it is still a partnership of sorts. Your donor will have his own questions and concerns, and may want to check you out just as much as you want to check him out. As in any parenting situation, your child's interests will be best served by this partnership working well.

You need to remember that—as things stand at the moment—a known donor may be able to obtain rights and responsibilities in relation to your child regardless of what you may want, and regardless of what you may have agreed. While he might be happy to give up all claims to the child before it is born, he may well change his mind when a real life little person appears, or when that real life little person becomes cute and fun and big enough to kick a footy around the park.

Many people are happy to have some involvement from a known donor. They see it as a good thing, a chance for their child to have a positive male role-model in their lives, another person who will love and care for them. The bottom line is, if you really don't want any involvement from the donor, your only guarantee is to use the protection of a clinic and choose an anonymous or identity-release donor.

> When we talked about parenting (with our donor dads) how one might bring up a child, what our roles would be—there were no issues on which we had major disagreement. We weren't getting any signals from them that there were going to be any major problems.
>
> Kris

Rights, roles and responsibilities

There are no rules, of course, about how and when to ask someone if they want to be a sperm donor. You know him best and you will pick the right time and place. You will probably want to do it with some degree of privacy to give him time to think it over. If he's still interested a week after you've asked, maybe you can invite him over

What we came to, I suppose, was that we had shifted through the pregnancy and first few months of his birth. We had always wanted the dads to be involved and that got stronger. I imagined that once Alfred was at school each of us would be home one day a week when he got home from school, and on Friday nights we'd all have dinner together. Having four parents makes it possible to provide a really good level of care whilst we're all still working, and can provide him with a really good family environment.

Kris

If you are going to have a known donor obviously you have to be very careful who that donor is. Someone once said to me, you have to assume that you all might completely change your mind once the baby is born. No matter what people say beforehand, that doesn't mean they'll feel like that afterwards. In the situation where the donor says, 'That's fine I'll go away. I won't want to be involved', women actually have to assume that he will change his mind. We were open to having the donors involved, so if they suddenly said we want more involvement we would have been happy with that, or at least not threatened by it.

Miranda

for dinner, crack open a bottle of wine and begin the discussion. The following list of questions is long but probably still not exhaustive and it might help you get started.

- What kind of family do you want to create?
- Is the role of the donor purely to donate sperm or will he and the child have an ongoing relationship?
- What will be the nature of that relationship?
- Will your donor be expected to play a role in the daily care and upbringing of the child?

- Will the donor be expected to be around as a support?
- Will the donor have any say in the big issues such as where you live, what religion the child will follow, what type of school they'll go to?
- Will the donor baby-sit, come to birthday parties, go to parent/teacher nights, buy Christmas presents, take the child on outings?
- Will contact between you be on a daily, weekly, or occasional basis?
- What happens if the donor decides he wants more access than you agreed?
- What happens he if decides he wants less?
- Will your donor have or seek any legal responsibilities towards the child?
- Will you identify him on the birth certificate?
- How might this affect any welfare government payments you are entitled to? How might it affect your tax?
- What happens if your child has an accident and you and your partner aren't around?
- What happens if one or both of you die while the child is still a dependent?
- Where will you all live?
- What if your donor or you wants to move interstate or overseas?
- Will he be expected to make a financial contribution to the maintenance of the child?
- Will this be a regular, fixed amount or an ad hoc arrangement? How will it be organised?
- Will he buy the pushchair or the cot, or pay for a month's nappy service?
- Will you expect your child to have a claim on his estate if he dies?
- Will your child be included in the donor's will or in any insurance policies or superannuation?
- How will you explain the relationship of the donor to your child when the time comes?
- What will the donor be called—the donor, your father, Dad, David?

- Will your donor's name be reflected in your child's name somewhere?
- Who will choose the child's first and/or middle names?
- Who are you going to tell about the donor and what are you going to tell them?
- Will you involve the donor's extended family?
- What relationship will your child have with the other set of uncles, aunts, cousins and grandparents?
- What happens if there is a relationship breakdown—if you split with your partner or he with his?
- What happens when a new person comes onto the scene?
- What happens if your donor marries or has other children?
- Will there be a relationship with those half siblings or will the two families stay completely separate?

We scheduled a time to get together and have a conversation [with the donors] and then we had several hours of discussion mostly around the roles we would all play and about parenting. We decided to write an agreement which included something about our roles and who would be the primary caregivers. We all acknowledged that it wouldn't be legally binding, but that we still thought it would be a good idea because it made us focus on some of the things we needed to think about. The agreement is funny . . . it's a mix of some quite technical legal bits and some wishy washy stuff about how we're starting off on this wonderful venture to create a new family.

Miranda

There was a lot in this initial agreement that was for further discussion—a lot of the agreement says we will keep talking about this. We recognised that until you have a child you actually can't know a lot of things about how you are going to feel.

Miranda

> We seem able to have these conversations, even when they [the donor couple] raise difficult issues. We are able to keep discussing things and I think that's the most important thing. They are very respectful of us and our position in relation to Alfred and we are trying to be respectful of them too. I see the whole thing as communication; we've got 20 years of communication ahead.
>
> Miranda

These are not simple issues to talk about and may be quite a challenge for everyone involved. The problem is, if you don't discuss them before there is a baby, you might find yourselves in trouble when there is. Certainly, you won't cover everything in your first discussion, and you will need to go away, think about what's been said, talk to other people, and then come back together to discuss it further. You don't need to make hard and fast decisions about these issues, but everyone involved needs to know they are at least thinking along the same lines. Above all, you need to clarify expectations about each person's role, rights and responsibilities. It is just not a good idea to go into an arrangement like this without everyone being clear where they stand.

You need to remember, too, that people change—jobs, partners and priorities—and becoming a parent can change people significantly. You might find that when there is a baby on the scene that either you, or your donor, feel differently about some of the things you've discussed. If you've established a good level of communication, and are used to talking things through, you will be far more able to deal with these changing expectations in a healthy and productive way. Your donor may decide, for example, he actually wants more involvement, and is already planning fishing trips and camping weekends or trips to the city or its equivalent, or maybe his parents have decided they like the idea of a grandchild and want to come over for Sunday tea. Alternatively, it might just all be too difficult for him—or for his partner—and even the agreed minimal level of contact is too much. Whatever the issue, it is important for your child's well-being that you have the mechanisms in place to deal with these ongoing changes.

After you've had all these discussion with your donor it is a good idea to write down what you have agreed—even if what you've agreed is that some things remain open and will require further discussion in the future. This agreement cannot be legally binding in any way, but it provides an opportunity for everyone involved to clarify their expectations. It can include all the big issues like where the child will live, who is expected to be the primary caregiver, what level of contact is expected between the child and the donor, what everybody's financial responsibilities are and what the child will be told. If everything does go horribly wrong between you and your donor and you end up in the Family Court, the agreement can be used to help demonstrate the intentions of everyone involved.

For all these reasons, using someone you contact over the Internet, or someone who responds to an advertisement, or someone you know only very superficially, is a risky option. There are just too many unknowns, too many things you cannot anticipate, too many things you cannot control. It just doesn't make much sense to involve a virtual stranger in something so hugely important, something over which, if he chose, he could exercise significant legal rights. If this is your only option, be cautious and try get to know the person over time, and find out as much as possible about them before you proceed.

Having said all that, there are many single women and lesbians couples who have used known donors and successfully negotiated good ongoing relationships where everyone is happy with the level of involvement, and the kids benefit from having a variety of people in their lives who love and look after them. There is no reason why, with some thought and planning, you shouldn't be able to use a known donor safely and successfully. Once you get to the stage of having an interested prospective donor—with whom you have covered all the groundwork —you can start to look at the medical issues involved.

> Our donors were screened and tested. They had tests periodically—initially in the early stages, then again before the insemination. They went to their doctor and said, 'This is what we want to do. What tests should we have?' They sent us copies of the results, and we also talked to them about their relationship and they said they were monogamous. We talked to them together. It may not be true, but we trusted them. They're pretty clean living boys.
>
> Miranda

> Before I decided, I got him to do the tests. I asked him to organise it. He went to his own doctor and got tested for HIV and Hepatitis B and C and also had a sperm count done because I didn't want to try with someone who had a low sperm count. And then I asked for copies of the results.
>
> Darcy

Health issues relating to the donor

There is a range of medical factors you and your donor need to consider in order to ensure his sperm is healthy and safe. This will involve talking about some fairly personal and intimate stuff, including his past and current sexual practices, and will also involve his undergoing a range of medical tests. Your primary concern should be to ensure there are no hereditary or infectious diseases that can be passed from the donor to you or your child via the semen. Once you have established this, you may also want to do a semen analysis to find out whether his sperm is healthy and has a good chance of fertilising your eggs. You will need to check out your donor's:

- family background, including any history of genetic or inherited illnesses (including mental illness)
- personal medical history, including any past sexually transmitted diseases and his current health status, including HIV and Hepatitis B and C

- current lifestyle, including safe-sex practices and any recreational drug use
- sperm quality and whether he has a low sperm count.

Family medical history

You will want to be confident that your donor does not have a family history of any genetic disorders that may be passed onto your child. Though many of these are relatively uncommon, it is worth checking just to be sure. They include haemophilia, Huntington's disease, cystic fibrosis, thalassemia, sickle cell anaemia and Tay Sachs disease. It may also be worth checking if you have recessive genes of any of these conditions yourself so that you can decide how vigilant you need to be with your donor. You might also want to establish whether there has been any history of genetic causes of intellectual disability, including Fragile X Syndrome, any serious mental illness, including bipolar disorder (manic depression) and schizophrenia, and any history of drug addiction or alcoholism.

Personal medical history and current health status

There are a number of infectious diseases that can be passed on to you and your baby via donor semen. These include gonorrhoea, chlamydia, syphilis, hepatitis B, HIV and cytomegalovirus (CMV). There is a chance of transmission of hepatitis C via insemination of semen, though this is very small. Your donor should undergo tests for all these. The tests can be performed by a local GP or at a men's health clinic, or at a specialised sexually transmitted diseases clinic.

The test for gonorrhoea and chlamydia is either by a penile swab or a urine sample. The test should be performed a minimum of two weeks after the last unsafe sexual contact to ensure the infection is detected. The test for hepatitis B, syphilis and HIV is by a blood test performed a minimum of three months after the last unsafe sexual contact, unsafe intravenous drug use or occupational exposure. (It is possible to be infected with these diseases, and for that infection not to show up in the first three months immediately afterwards.)

Cytomegalovirus (CMV) is a herpes virus that can be transmitted via semen from a man who is CMV antibody positive to a woman who is CMV antibody negative. The risk to the foetus if the mother does become infected is significant, although the chances of this infection happening are very small. An antibody positive person can occasionally become infectious when the virus reactivates, and during this time the virus can be shed into the semen. There is currently no reliable method of testing the semen to determine whether the man is shedding CMV, and sperm washing techniques are not reliable as a screening mechanism. If the woman is infected while she is pregnant it can lead to severe abnormalities in the baby, similar to those caused by rubella, or to miscarriage. It is possible, however, for the woman to be tested periodically during the inseminations to ensure she has not caught the virus.

Lifestyle and safe-sex practices

If your donor tests negative to all the above, and if there has been no possibility of exposure to any infectious disease for three months prior to the tests, his semen should be safe to use for an insemination. One of the problems with using fresh semen from a known donor, however, is that you need to be confident that the semen remains safe over time. This means that your donor must abstain from any unsafe practices, including unprotected sex or shared needles, for the whole time you are inseminating. If he does not continue safe practices, there will be a risk of infection to you and your baby.

For most men—and hopefully for your donor—this will not be a problem at all, but for others it may be an issue. It is really important, however, that you have this discussion with your donor however difficult it might be—you can always start by lending him this book! If you are lucky, you might fall pregnant in the first six months, but you could just as easily find yourself inseminating for much longer. Your donor needs to be aware that this could be a long-term commitment, and that it may have an ongoing effect on his lifestyle. One possible solution to this may be to freeze your donor's sperm at an infertility clinic, though this is not available everywhere (see below).

Semen analysis

If your donor has fathered children before, the chances are that his sperm is healthy and fully functioning—though there is still no guarantee of this, especially if he had kids a long time ago. If he has never fathered a child, you will not know how healthy his sperm is. Approximately 10 per cent of men have a problem with their sperm that can affect their capacity to father a child. It is possible to get your donor's sperm checked before you use it by having a semen analysis (see Chapter 1) done at an infertility clinic or through a local GP.

You may decide that the chances of there being a problem are pretty low and that you really don't want to go to the time, inconvenience and additional expense of having a semen analysis done. On the other hand, you might feel that it is worth the extra effort to be confident that the donor sperm you are using has every chance of fertilising your eggs. There have certainly been instances of women using a known donor without success and—after some time—having the sperm analysed only to discover there was something wrong with it, and there was never any chance of their conceiving. If you decide not to do a sperm analysis in the first instance, it might be worth doing one if you have not conceived after, say, six months. You certainly don't want to go through a year or so of trying, only to have to start all over again with a new donor because of low sperm numbers or poor motility of your original donor's sperm.

There are some additional health and lifestyle factors that are known to affect the quality of sperm (see Chapter 2). These include smoking, using various prescription and non-prescription drugs, including marijuana, and exposure to toxins or chemicals. You need to bear these things in mind when making an assessment of whether there might be anything wrong with your donor's sperm. Certainly, a good level of general health all round is an advantage.

Medical issues related to the prospective biological mother

The medical considerations for a prospective mother are the same whether you are single or married, lesbian or straight (see Chapters 1 and 2). You should have a pap smear and breast examination, check your rubella immunity and have another vaccination if necessary. If you do have a rubella vaccination you then need to wait three months before you begin inseminating. In consultation with your doctor, you should assess the chances of your having contracted any sexually transmitted diseases in the past. If you think there is a risk of this, you need to get tested and treated appropriately. You might want to get your blood pressure checked, find out your blood group and whether you have any antibodies in your blood, and make sure you are not anaemic. You might also want to check for common recessive genetic conditions.

Tracking ovulation

The inseminations need to be performed at your fertile time—that is, when your egg is released from the ovary at ovulation (see Chapter 3). Most women who have regular 28-day cycles ovulate around mid cycle—that is, on about day 14 (day 1 is the first day of your period). The problem is, however, that many women ovulate before or after day 14, or might ovulate on day 14 one month, and then on day 16 the next, and on day 15 the one after that. If you have a short cycle—26 days—or a long cycle—32 days—your ovulation may be different again. In order to conceive you have to get the timing right. You should start by keeping close track of when your periods come and making a note of the dates over, say, three or four cycles. You can then start to track your ovulation each month. There are a number of ways to do this (see Chapter 1).

If you have very irregular periods and you really can't seem to find any pattern to your cycles at all, it might be worth seeing a specialist to see if there is something wrong with your ovulation (see Chapter 4).

When to do the inseminations

The inseminations need to be performed at your fertile time—that is, at ovulation. You are most fertile immediately before ovulation and on the day of ovulation. Your egg is able to be fertilised for approximately 12 to 24 hours and the sperm can last up to two or three days inside you. You may maximise your chances of conceiving by inseminating as close as possible to ovulation, and by doing more than one insemination. You may want to do the first insemination one to two days prior to ovulation, and the second on the actual day of ovulation. If you have ample sperm you can do a third, the following day. It is difficult to be exact and there is certainly an element of luck involved. If you inseminate a couple of times, around ovulation, you should have a good chance of the egg and sperm being in the right place at the right time.

Unless you can be confident that you are ovulating, and you can identify the time with reasonable accuracy, there's not much point in trying self insemination.

> While I was searching for a donor I was getting to know my body in detail. I knew when my cycles were. I knew my temperature changes. I knew when I ovulated. I knew how many days my periods were. I was very regular. I had a pattern. I did three inseminations: pre-ovulation, ovulation and post ovulation. He would come and I had all the equipment and he would deposit in a jar and I would do it. I made sure I had an orgasm because that helps. I ended up doing that for about a year, every month.
>
> Darcy

How to do the inseminations

The best way to do the inseminations is to have your donor produce the semen at the same place that you do the insemination. If this is

> Initially, we were doing the inseminations as part of our sexual relationship, but as time went on it became harder to do that and it's actually not the best thing for your sex life. You're not really focused on enjoying sex, and in the end it was better just to do the inseminations.
>
> Kris

not possible, the donor must make sure he keeps the semen warm and gets it to you within an hour of ejaculating. The sperm is at its best for the first 20 minutes or so and starts to deteriorate after about an hour. Your donor should ejaculate into a plastic or glass container which must be clean, but does not need to be sterile. It is important that the first part of the ejaculate—which contains the most sperm—gets into the container. He should avoid using any type of lubricant as most are toxic to sperm.

Despite the enduring image of the 'turkey baster', this is not actually the best tool for the job. Most women use a standard plastic 5 millimetre syringe which you can buy over the counter at a chemist. If you feel awkward asking for one—or if the pharmacist asks you what it's for—you can always say it's for giving medicine to a child. Draw the semen up into the syringe, place it gently in the vagina, and squeeze the syringe until all the semen is inserted. You can do this yourself, or your partner can do it. It is probably best done with you lying on your back with your hips slightly tilted. Once the semen has been inserted, it is important to remain in this position—with a pillow supporting your hips if necessary—for about half an hour. After that you can get up and go about your normal daily business.

There is some evidence to suggest that having an orgasm immediately before or after the insemination may help. When you have an orgasm, the cervix opens slightly which may encourage the sperm to head off in the right direction towards the egg. Some lesbian couples like to make the insemination part of a sexual experience anyway, or to do something that makes it more intimate, or that involves the non-biological mother. Some women like to create an atmosphere by playing music, using candles or soft lighting, or having some kind of ceremony—especially the first time. Other women have found that, because the focus is on the insemination, the sexual part doesn't actually work well, and they prefer to keep the two things separate. You might also find, however, that after the third, forth or fifth attempt, the intimacy falls by the wayside and the procedure becomes a little more perfunctory.

Pregnancy test

You can do a pregnancy test a day or two after your next missed period. The urine tests you buy from the chemists are generally pretty accurate. If there is any ambiguity—if you test positive but still get your period, for example (see Chapter 4)—you may want to do another test a week later, or see your local GP for a blood test. If the result is negative, you need to start tracking your ovulation again in preparation for the next insemination.

To have a realistic chance of getting pregnant through straightforward donor insemination, you probably need to try at least half a dozen times, and many women will try considerably more than this. There is certainly an element of luck here, but your sexual and medical history and your general health may affect your chances, and your age certainly will. In any one attempt there is roughly a 15 to 20 per cent chance of conceiving.

Depending on your particular circumstances you might want to think about seeing a GP or a gynaecologist after six to eight unsuccessful attempts, just to make sure there is nothing obviously wrong with your fertility. If you haven't had an analysis done of your donor's semen, it is worth getting that done now. After this, you might want to continue trying for longer with him, or you might think about using a different donor. At some stage, you might want to talk to a specialist at an infertility clinic with a view to having some low-key medical intervention.

Using a clinic donor

You may choose to approach an infertility clinic for help if you have done a number of unsuccessful inseminations with a known donor that have not been successful, or if you can't find a donor, or if you do not want to use a known donor. Many women prefer to use a clinic because the sperm donor is screened and they know the sperm is completely safe, or because they don't want any personal involvement with a donor, or because they are reluctant to place a friend in a difficult legal position. Whether you can use a clinic, however, will depend on where you live.

Legal status of state clinics

Access to infertility treatment services for single women and lesbians varies from state to state. In Victoria, South Australia and Western Australia, there is specific legislation governing assisted reproductive technology that determines who can legally access services. In New South Wales, Queensland, Tasmania, Northern Territory and Australian Capital Territory, there is no specific legislation. Where there is no legislation, clinics generally work to guidelines set down by the National Health and Medical Research Council, and are directed by their own ethics committees.

Detailed below is the current legal situation in each state or territory. The legislation is being challenged and changed all the time, however, and although this information is correct at the time of going to press, you should always call your local clinic directly to check whether any changes have occurred.

Victoria

In Victoria assisted reproductive treatment is governed by the *Infertility Treatment Act 1995* and through the Infertility Treatment Authority, the statutory body that administers the legislation. Currently, fertile single woman and lesbians cannot access any donor sperm for insemination services. This means that a clinic cannot inseminate a woman with her own known donor sperm, or screen or freeze that sperm, or provide her with anonymous or identity-release donor sperm. This may change in the future.

A clinic can provide information and advice, undertake testing and provide preliminary treatments that don't involve sperm—for example, monitoring your periods and helping you work out your ovulation, or prescribing treatment to regulate your ovulation. Some interstate clinics are affiliated with Victorian clinics, which means you can have part of your treatment at home—tracking ovulation, blood tests, ultrasound scans and injections—and then travel interstate for the inseminations.

A single woman or lesbian can, however, access in vitro fertilisation (IVF) treatment in Victoria if she is deemed 'medically infertile'. Whether or not you are 'medically infertile' is determined by a specialist who will undertake a clinical evaluation which will normally include an exploratory laparoscopy. If you do not have a pre-existing condition that renders you 'medically infertile' you will have to travel interstate for at least six cycles of donor insemination and, if after those six attempts, you are still not pregnant, you can arrange to see a fertility specialist in Victoria. That specialist will take into account your age and medical history—including the six unsuccessful cycles—and may deem you medically infertile. You can then access IVF treatment in Victoria, but not donor insemination. This leaves many women with a difficult choice between continuing low-key inseminations interstate, or getting full IVF treatment at home. All donor sperm used in Victoria for any procedure is identity-release.

South Australia

In South Australia infertility treatment is governed by the *Reproductive Technology Act 1988*, and through the South Australian Council on Reproductive Technology. The situation in South Australia is currently very similar to that of Victoria. Fertile single women and lesbians cannot access donor sperm for self-insemination or insemination by a clinic. The only option for women wanting donor insemination is to travel interstate. You can access infertility treatment if you are 'medically infertile' but, again, this means IVF, not donor insemination. If you have some pre-existing condition or, if after six attempts of donor insemination you are still not successful, you can arrange to see a specialist in South Australia who will determine whether or not you are medically infertile. In determining this the specialist will take into account your age and medical history, as well as the six unsuccessful cycles. If you are deemed medically infertile you can then access IVF using donor sperm. Donor sperm is non-identity release—that is, anonymous, although some clinics have set up voluntary registers.

Western Australia

Infertility treatment in Western Australia is governed by the *Human Reproductive Technology Act 1991* and through the Reproductive Technology Council. Certain amendments were recently made to this legislation, however, by the *Acts Amendment (Lesbian and Gay Law Reform Bill 2001)*. As a result of this bill, single women and lesbians can access the full range of donor insemination services and IVF treatment.

Sperm from known donors can be screened and frozen and will be released for use after being quarantined for six months. Known donors are required to go through a medical screening process and answer a detailed lifestyle questionnaire—similar to that required of blood donors—but are not automatically barred if they are gay. If you do not have, or prefer not to use, a known donor, you can access anonymous donor sperm. If donor insemination is unsuccessful, you can proceed to IVF treatment at any stage you and your doctor feel appropriate.

Currently, all donors recruited by the clinic are anonymous, non-identity release. Identifying information is held on a central register and can be released if all parties agree, but neither the donor recipient nor child have automatic access to the information.

New South Wales

Single women and lesbians can access the full range of donor insemination services and IVF treatment in New South Wales. Known donor sperm can be used after screening, but gay donors will be excluded. There is likely to be a six-month quarantine period on the sperm. There are no restrictions on the use of anonymous donor sperm, though not all clinics have donor sperm available. Currently, the sperm that is available is from anonymous donors and is not identity release. The clinic may contact the donor on behalf of the recipient or the recipient's child to access further non-identifying or medical information, but will not release any identifying information. There are moves to change this, however, to a formal identity-release model. If donor insemination doesn't work you can proceed to IVF.

Tasmania

It is possible for single women and lesbians to access the full range of donor insemination services and IVF treatment in Tasmania, though currently only one clinic provides access to donor sperm. You can use your own known donor or anonymous donor sperm. Prospective donors have to undergo screening and complete a lifestyle questionnaire, but are not automatically excluded if they are gay. Sperm from known donors has to be quarantined for six months before it can be used. Currently, donors are only accepted if they agree to provide identifying information which may later be released to the child of the recipient.

Queensland

It is possible for single women and lesbians to access the full range of donor insemination services and IVF treatment in Queensland, though not all clinics provide services to lesbians and single women—clinics can legally discriminate against you, but not all do. You can use your own known donor or an anonymous donor. Where a known donor is used, he is required to undergo screening and complete a detailed lifestyle questionnaire. It is likely that he will be excluded if he is gay. Where the donor is accepted there is a six-month quarantine period on the sperm. You can, however, access anonymous donor sperm and have your inseminations done at the clinic. If donor insemination is unsuccessful, you can proceed to IVF treatment. Whether the sperm is anonymous or identity-release will vary from donor to donor and clinic to clinic as there are no overriding regulations. You may be able to ask for an identity-release donor, but this will depend on the individual clinic, and on what sperm is currently available.

Australian Capital Territory

Single women and lesbians can access the full range of donor insemination services and IVF treatment in the ACT. You can use your own known donor or an anonymous donor. Where a known donor is used, he is required to go through the medical screening process and complete a detailed lifestyle questionnaire. A donor will not automatically be barred from donating sperm because he is gay. The donor sperm is usually held in quarantine for six months, but in some circumstances it may be possible to waive the quarantine period. All sperm provided by the clinic used is completely anonymous and no identifying information can be given to the donor recipient or the child of the recipient without the express consent of the donor. If you have no success getting pregnant using donor insemination you can proceed to IVF treatment when appropriate.

Northern Territory

Currently, there is no access to infertility treatment services for lesbians and single women in the Northern Territory. Although there is no legislation barring the provision of services to single women and lesbians, the contract between the Northern Territory Government and the clinic restricts the provision of such services to married couples and de facto heterosexual couples who have been together for three years. The clinic requires evidence of this in the form of a marriage certificate or statutory declaration. This restriction is currently being challenged but, while it stands, the only way for lesbians and single women to access treatment is to travel interstate.

Finding a supportive clinic

If you have a choice of clinics—or if you are going to have to travel interstate—it is certainly worth doing some research before you make an appointment. In addition to getting a general sense of the clinic (see Chapter 1) you will want to get an idea of how single or lesbian friendly it is. As a general rule, avoid any that have religious affiliations; it is unlikely they will provide services to you. Ask around your social circle and/or talk to someone who has had treatment. You might be able to get a recommendation from a supportive GP or health centre, or you could try a local prospective parenting group (see Information and resources).

Once you have the name of a clinic, call them and see what kind of response you get. You can ask them directly whether they provide services to single women and lesbians, and how long they have been providing those services. If they've been doing it for a while, they will be more accommodating when you turn up on your own, or with your partner. Ask them how many donors they have available to single women and lesbians and whether they are anonymous or identity-release. Once you've found a clinic that sounds okay, you will need to get a referral from your GP and make an appointment. Wherever you go for treatment you will have a consultation with a specialist and a counsellor before you can access any services.

> After the first consultation we were required to see a counsellor. It was just the two of us having an informal chat with the counsellor. It was quite useful and it covered all the topics that were relevant having a non-standard family arrangement, our motivation for wanting to have children, and issues around donors as well. It was not like some form of interrogation. It didn't feel invasive. It felt realistic. You know, 'Have you thought about all these things?' And you ought to be able to say, 'Yes I have.' It was reasonably supportive and I thought it was useful.
>
> Maria

Supplying your own donor

If you have concerns about the safety of your known donor sperm, or if you want to freeze your sperm, it might be worth thinking about approaching an infertility clinic. You and your donor will both need to see a doctor who will ask preliminary questions about your medical/fertility history and you will need to see a counsellor who will explain how the screening process and freezing works. Your donor will be tested for a variety of genetic and infectious diseases and will have to provide a semen sample for analysis. The sperm will then be frozen and quarantined for six months. At the end of that six months the donor will be tested again. If he tests negative for any infectious diseases, the sperm will be released to you. You then track your ovulation and have the insemination done at the appropriate time.

Insemination procedure

The insemination is performed by a doctor or nurse at the clinic. The procedure is very similar to having a pap smear. You will be asked to undress from the waist down, step up onto a bed and lie

> The first insemination was a bit traumatic, not having been through a procedure like that before, other than a pap smear. The level of discomfort was similar to a pap smear but psychologically it was worse, more stressful. There was no pain, just unpleasantness. It was fine after that though. After that first one I actually preferred to do it on my own. I just thought of it as a straightforward medical procedure—low key, no big deal—and that made it easier.
>
> Jacki

on your back with your legs slightly apart. The doctor or nurse will then insert a speculum. They will either insert the sperm directly into the vagina with a plastic syringe, or will insert a catheter connected to the syringe through the speculum and through your cervix and insert the sperm into your uterus. Both procedures should only take a few minutes. Most women do not find them painful, but for some women they can be. If it does hurt, ask the doctor or nurse to stop. It does help to relax, but this is easier said than done. Sometimes it can help if the doctor or nurse uses a smaller speculum. If it continues to be painful you can ask your doctor to give you something to help you relax. You should be able to get up and move about immediately afterwards.

Using a donor from the clinic

If you do not have your own donor, or if you prefer to use an anonymous donor, you will need to access donor sperm from a clinic. The advantage of this is that the semen is screened and you can be confident it is completely safe. Also, you do not have to enter into any of the complex negotiations about shared parenting that you have to with a known donor and the legal situation relating to the donor is very clear.

You will need to see the clinic doctor, and are required to attend a session with a counsellor. Counselling is standard practice and is required in all situations where donor gametes are used. Counselling provides you with an opportunity to explore the issues involved in using an anonymous or identity-release donor, to find out exactly how everything works and to ask questions about things that are unclear. The counsellor should also explain to you what donors they have available and provide you with their profiles.

Well I guess the idea of having kids has always been there, part of the life plan since my teenage years. We had some friends who had investigated all the options for donor insemination and it seemed like it was possible to do. We were quite comfortable using an anonymous donor because it seemed like a less complex arrangement, not having a third party involved.

Jacki

We thought there may have been problems using a known donor, to do with the rights of the child and the rights of the donor. There are a lot of issues using a known donor and I think it can be rather fraught and more complex than people think.

Maria

Donor profiles

Clinics vary in the information they provide about each donor. You can expect to be provided with details about a range of physical characteristics, including height, weight, build, ethnic background, and hair, eye and skin colour. You can also expect to be told the donor's age and whether he has fathered other children. In some

Of course, there are disadvantages for the child using a non-identity release donor, but that was the only thing available to us. We are hopeful that the rules may change in the future and, maybe, it'll be possible to approach the donor. As we have gone through the process our awareness of the issues around using anonymous and identity-release donors has increased and perhaps now we feel a bit more strongly about having access to identifying information about the donor than we did at the beginning. It seems like a fairer option for the child if they can find out.

Jacki

We had a choice of three donors: a real estate agent, a masseur and a music student. That was pretty much the extent of the information available, except for basic physical characteristics—height, weight, hair colour, etc. Out of the three none seemed any more suited than the other . . . apart from our prejudices against the real estate agent! The masseur had dark skin and a heavy build, so we went with the medium-built music student. In an ideal world you wouldn't have to go interstate for treatment, and you would have more options for donors. I'm not suggesting you need a thousand people to choose from, but three was pretty tricky.

Maria

I guess the other problem with the limited number of donors is that if a substantial proportion of the clientele using these donors are lesbians travelling interstate, that's a relatively small community, and that could get difficult. So far no one else has mentioned donor number 438! You've just got to remember your number!

Jacki

cases the donor profile may include information about the age at which his parents and grandparents died and their cause of death. The profile may also include details of minor medical problems, including wearing glasses or having allergies. Some profiles include information about the donor's educational background, his qualifications, job, and personal interests. Some even include comments on why he has decided to donate sperm and a general statement to the recipient.

Different people will be more and less influenced by different aspects of the profile. You might want the child to have the same basic colouring as you, or you might be more interested in the donor's education level, or by the comments he makes about why he is donating. It is also possible that you may start with one donor whose sperm supply runs out, so you will need to choose another. If you've done a few cycles with one donor that haven't been successful, you might want to try another donor anyway. If you conceive with a particular donor, you may want to use that donor again for a second child. For single women and lesbian couples, having the same donor means the children share the same biological background. For lesbian couples where both partners want to have a child, using the same donor means that the children will be biologically related through the donor. Some clinics may allow you to buy a supply of your donor's sperm to freeze with a view to using later, but because of the general shortage of sperm, this is not always possible. They might also be willing to contact the donor to ask him for more sperm. These things are generally negotiated on an individual basis.

Once you have seen the doctor and counsellor and selected a donor you will need to monitor your ovulation and attend the clinic at a specific time for your doctor to perform the insemination (see above). If you are having your insemination done interstate, you should be able to arrange to have any monitoring—blood tests and scan—and any trigger injections done locally. This means that you should only have to make one trip to your interstate clinic.

> We were quite keen to have the same donor for our second child as it seemed to offer some advantages down the track, particularly in our situation where we have a non-identity release donor. If the children want to find their father, at least if they have the same father, they have the same search. It would be more difficult if you had the situation where one child had access to their father and the other didn't. That would be a very difficult family situation to be in. It is fairer to have them both on an even footing.
>
> Jacki

Supply of donor sperm

In Australia at the moment there is a very limited supply of donor sperm. Unlike other countries—most notably North America—it is illegal to pay for sperm (although donors are generally paid 'expenses'), and most donors here do it for altruistic reasons. Some donors may be reluctant to donate because of the increasing trend towards identification. Some clinics allow donors to specify who their sperm goes to, which means single women and lesbians sometimes miss out. Not all clinics allow this, however. The effect of all this is that you may have access to only a handful of donors, and in some cases only one or two.

You might want to check with the counsellor about how many other women are using these donors. With so few available, you need to be aware that it is possible your child will have a number of biological half-siblings. Each donor is normally used for a maximum of ten families, which means there may be ten or more half-siblings. In reality, donors come and go, and may not be around long enough to be responsible for this many children. For lesbians, given the closeness of the community, it is also possible you might know other women who are using the same donor. This is not necessarily a problem, but it is something about which you should be aware.

Medical checks

If you've done a few cycles of donor insemination—either at home or at a clinic—without success, you might want to think about getting some help from an infertility specialist. At what stage you do this will depend upon your particular circumstances and priorities. Some women are reluctant to get doctors involved at all and would rather keep trying for a year or so; others are quite happy to receive some low-key medical intervention early on. If you are over 35, or have problems with your periods and/or ovulation, or suspect you may have a problem resulting from a sexually transmitted disease, you might want to get yourself checked out sooner rather than later.

An infertility specialist can check that your hormone levels are normal and that you are ovulating. They can monitor your ovulation with blood tests and ultrasound scans and make sure the inseminations are being performed at exactly the right time. They can give you drugs to regulate your cycle, or to make you produce more eggs so that your chances of conceiving are higher. They can suggest a range of exploratory procedures (see Chapter 1) if they think you may have a problem with blocked tubes, or endometriosis, or something else that may be affecting your fertility such as an infection. If you are having problems conceiving, seeing a specialist at this stage might make all the difference.

Further options for treatment—IVF

If you have tried donor insemination for some time and, even with some medical assistance, you have been unsuccessful in getting pregnant, you may want to try a cycle of IVF. Statistically, you have a slightly better chance of conceiving with IVF than with donor insemination. IVF, of course, is a much bigger deal, involving a much greater level of medical intervention and higher costs. Certainly, it might not be what you expected you would be doing when you started trying to get pregnant. It's a big step and will require a lot of thought and discussion before you proceed. If you are part of a couple, another option might be to change roles—that is, the other partner tries donor insemination. This will depend on a whole range of personal and medical factors, however, and may not be an option for all couples.

If you do proceed to IVF, the only real difference between you and most heterosexual couples, is that the sperm you use will come from a donor, not from your partner. Otherwise the process is exactly the same (see Chapter 6).

> It is quite emotionally difficult [doing donor insemination] even at that low level of medical intervention—or no medical intervention—when there's a constant lack of success. I just got to the point where I thought, well the next step for me is a laparoscopy and I didn't want to go down that track straightaway so instead we decided Miranda would start trying.
>
> Kris

Importing sperm from overseas

In some states it is possible to buy and import sperm from sperm banks overseas. You can select from a wide range of donors and can access a lot of information about those donors. A catalogue can be mailed to you or you can access it online. You must be registered with a clinic in Australia, which will receive and store the sperm. Importing sperm is, however, quite complicated and very expensive. While the cost of the actual sperm is similar to here, the shipping costs for a cryro-preservation container are considerable. Whether or not you can do it will also depend on the laws and regulations governing the release of information about the donor in the state in which you live. In some cases, because the overseas clinics are unwilling to allow identifying information to be released to the Australian clinic—even though they agree to the information being released to the child at a later date—the Australian clinic cannot legally use the sperm. Also, there have been situations where a person has bought and imported sperm into one state and, when they later transferred to another state for further treatment, they have not been able to transfer the sperm with them. In South Australia, Victoria and New South Wales you cannot import sperm without the express permission from the respective regulatory body. You will need to discuss all this with your local clinic.

I had to deal with Miranda getting pregnant on her second try [after I'd tried for quite a while]. It was a weird combination actually, because I was kind of ecstatic that she was pregnant, but I was a bit upset it wasn't me and I wondered whether it would ever be me. I was a bit jealous I guess. I had a couple of days and I got over it pretty quickly and started focusing on the baby.

Kris

As a fertile single woman not able to be treated in Victoria, my only choice of donor sperm was non-identity release from a clinic in New South Wales. My first big dilemma was that I didn't want that sperm. I contacted America and got all sorts of information from sperm banks and, in the end, purchased nine vials of sperm from there.

Wendy

Personal issues for lesbian couples

If you do end up having infertility treatment—especially IVF—as a lesbian couple, your experience may differ in some ways from that of heterosexual couples. There are certainly advantages and disadvantages for two women undergoing treatment, though obviously the medical side will be exactly the same.

You will undoubtedly have to deal with negative attitudes about your decision to have children, either from people close to you—colleagues, friends or family even—or from people further afield—social commentators, religious leaders, politicians, Joe public. Even with today's much greater levels of acceptance of lesbian and gay sexuality, the mention of children seems to bring out any latent homophobia. This can feel like a double whammy when you are struggling with infertility.

Going through treatment is tough enough at the best of times and, when you are feeling exhausted and teary after ten days of injections, you can do without the latest tabloid survey declaring how many people think you shouldn't have children. Attitudes are changing, however, and will continue to change as more and more lesbians and gay men become involved in parenting. Anecdotal evidence points to a 'lesbian baby boom', which will only make it easier in the future. There are a number of small, but active, lesbian parenting groups popping up everywhere who can provide support. Most include people who are trying to get pregnant, as well as those who already have kids.

Depending on where you live, you may experience problems in accessing services in the first place—some clinics, of course, still don't offer any services to lesbian couples—and you may have to travel long distances to a clinic that will actually treat you. Having treatment long distance is very difficult because of all the additional problems of transport, accommodation and negotiating time off work, and all the extra expense. Some clinics have been treating lesbian couples for a while and are fully lesbian-friendly, others are in the early stages of this process and staff might not be quite as supportive as you would like.

Some women have found that doctors tend to view them as single, that they don't really know how to treat their partner and that the partner ends up feeling sidelined. In other situations, doctors have assumed that because the partner in this case is a woman, she will understand exactly what her partner is going through, and be completely empathetic. To a degree, the partner may be able to identify with some aspects of the process—mood swings, period pain, internal examinations and speculums—but this is a long way from understanding the experience of infertility and going through treatment. Although the partner who is not having treatment may be very much involved in the process of creating this family, she has no social standing, or legal relationship to what's happening, and is less likely to be afforded the affirmation that normally comes with parenthood.

Many lesbian women who end up facing the possibility of IVF treatment do so because they have had a number of cycles of donor insemination which have been unsuccessful. Moving from donor insemination (DI) to IVF is a big step, and not everyone will take it. Whether you do or don't will depend on a whole range of personal factors, including how old you are, how many times you've tried DI, whether you're forced to travel interstate, whether one or both of you are trying, your financial situation and how much patience you have.

One of the significant advantages that two women have over heterosexual couples is that, theoretically, you have two chances of creating a family. Both partners may not want to try to conceive—age, careers, medical issues or just personal choice will affect this decision—but where both partners are happy to try, you have a better chance of eventually being a parent. If one partner is not successful with DI or with IVF, the other can try—you would be very unlucky for both of you to be infertile.

While changing the partner who has treatment because one is unable to conceive may be the answer in the long run, it can also present significant challenges. There is a whole range of practical and emotional issues to deal with, and it is not an easy decision to make. Will one partner stop completely or will you alternate cycles? What if there is some overlap and you both get pregnant at the same time? What is best for the children? What is best for your relationship? How will you manage the effects of back-to-back treatments? Will one partner stop as soon as the other conceives? What emotional effects might this have on both of you? How will you cope financially?

If one partner stops trying, she will still have to deal with her own possible infertility, her own feelings of grief and loss, even if she still ends up being a parent because her partner has a baby. She may still lose out on the pregnancy and on the experience of giving birth and breastfeeding. She may miss out on having a child who is genetically hers, who is related to her parents and siblings. If her partner gets pregnant pretty quickly, she might struggle to feel as positive as she would like to be.

She will likely be going through her own grieving process, and this can make it very difficult. She may be overjoyed at the thought of finally having a family and being a mum, but saddened that she is not the one to carry and have the baby. She might be relieved at having a good excuse to stop treatment, but disappointed that it didn't work for her. She may be happy and sad at the same time. Most women don't have to deal with their infertility at the same time as being in close proximity to someone who is pregnant. In fact, they generally go out of their way to avoid anything that reminds them of babies and birth. A lesbian who is a mum because her partner gave birth doesn't get to do this.

Her partner will want to be excited about her pregnancy and to share it, but may be wary about being too enthusiastic. It's a difficult situation for both partners. None of this is insurmountable, of course; it can be a happy and positive time for both. It may just take some open and honest communication and a little extra care and sensitivity. Those clinics in major urban centres that have been treating lesbians for a while may have counsellors who can help; smaller clinics in country areas will probably not.

Perhaps the other advantage for two women is that if one has problems getting pregnant, she can donate her eggs to her partner who might be able to successfully carry the child. This is completely legal where clinics use donor eggs or embryos. When a woman donates eggs, however, she gives up all legal rights to any child born from them. This means that, legally, the mother of the child is the partner who carries it and gives birth. Where this works it can be a very positive outcome for a couple as both have a biological connection to the child.

Personal issues for single women

Much of what applies to couples experiencing infertility is also relevant to single women. There are, however, some important differences in the experience of going through treatment on your own. Managing the practical side of treatment can be especially tough—finding someone who can do your injections, or pick you up after treatment, or take care of you after a procedure. There are many occasions during treatment where it helps to have a second person around.

> While I feel that I have been fortunate in that I did find someone to father my child, there is sadness in that he is not my partner, that he isn't sharing the day-to-day changes of development in James that I would like to share with a partner. In an ideal world I would like to share it with a partner. But I think I have been quite fortunate with my donor.
>
> Darcy

Whereas couples can share the burden of treatment, you have to deal with everything pretty much on your own. Even if you have a good support network of friends, it can still be difficult to share what can be an intensely personal experience, and you may sometimes feel

> During the actual procedures and the treatments I'm fine; I have my mum or my sister, usually, or sometimes a close friend. At other times though, I feel like I am doing all this alone, when I am at home by myself at night. I never wanted to be a single parent and there's a side of me that occasionally thinks, 'What the hell are you doing? This was not the plan'. But again, that desire not to go through life without children is just that much stronger than the, 'Oh my God, I'm doing this on my own'.
>
> Wendy

isolated. While there are numerous established support groups for heterosexual couples, and new, emerging ones for lesbian couples, there is no real equivalent for single women. Other single mums are not really in the same position, and will not necessarily have any understanding of what it is like to go through infertility. This can make it especially tough on days when you might just want to talk to someone else who understands what you are going through. There *are* other single women out there, though it might just be a bit more difficult to find them. The existing networks, or the clinics, should be able to put you in touch.

You may have already experienced a sense of loss from one or more personal relationships that have ended. You may be grieving the loss of a life-partner and the loss of dreams and expectations about how your life would turn out. Often this loss—like the loss of infertility—goes unacknowledged. Depending on where you live, you may have had problems getting treatment in the first place because of legal restrictions. You may also find yourself on the receiving end of negative comments about your choices in regard to personal relationships, or about choosing to be a single mum, either from people you know personally, or the media. Most women develop their own strategies for dealing with this, but it can still be hard when you are having to manage a whole range of issues regarding your infertility as well.

> If you're single, I think you need one or two levels of support—immediate family or a close friend or colleague . . . someone who knows you well enough so you can just blurt out absolutely anything and pretty much get the response you need at the time. Otherwise it would be really hard to manage, especially for any length of time. For me, there are three different areas: my home life (where I'm on my own), my work and my family. Because I get support from family and work it really helps when I am on my own. The support and conversations I have at work are very different from what I receive and what I want from my family. If you are single, try and find different avenues for support, because you have different emotions and needs at different times.
>
> Wendy

> I went to see my GP and told her I was thinking about getting pregnant, omitting the fact that I didn't have a partner. She was just like, 'Oh yes. That's lovely. You'll need a physical.' And I said, 'No. You don't understand. I'm not married.' And she said, 'Oh that's okay these days!'
>
> Wendy

Summing up

- There is a range of options available to single women and lesbians who want to have a child, though not all the options are available in all states and some women will have to travel interstate to access donor sperm or have donor inseminations.

- Where a single woman or lesbian uses donor sperm provided through a clinic there is no legal relationship between the donor and any child born from that donor's sperm. However, the legal relationship between a donor personally known to a single woman or lesbian and a child from that donor remains legally unclear.
- Using a known donor raises a number of complex personal, health and legal issues which are best managed by ongoing open and honest communication between the donor and the recipient. It is really important that everyone involved is clear about their rights, roles and responsibilities before proceeding with any inseminations.
- Both the prospective biological mother and the sperm donor should undergo certain basic health checks before proceeding with any inseminations. Inseminations can be done safely and privately at home using a variety of methods to monitor ovulation.
- Infertility clinics can provide advice and information about conception, and help with tracking your ovulation or investigating your general gynaecological health. Depending on where you live, you may also be able to access donor sperm and insemination services, and IVF treatment.
- There may be some additional or different personal issues for single women and lesbian couples trying donor insemination over an extended period of time, or undergoing IVF treatment.

8
How do you feel?
Responses to infertility and its treatment

Every individual's experience of infertility and its treatment is different. How you and your partner react will depend on a whole range of things, including the type of treatment you are having and how many cycles you do, how you respond physically to the treatment, how your body recovers between cycles, whether you have experienced repeated pregnancy loss, the nature of your relationship with your partner and the effectiveness of your support networks, your relationship with your doctor, your financial situation, your family background and personality, and other things that are going on in your life at the time.

If you conceive very quickly after one or two rounds of relatively straightforward treatment, and have an easy pregnancy and a healthy birth, the negative or lasting effects of your infertility and treatment will probably not be as bad as if you undergo complex treatment for many years with continual disappointment. It's not a competition, though, and any diagnosis of infertility is tough. Even one cycle of treatment can be difficult. No one dealing with infertility and its treatment finds it easy. Everyone has a story to tell.

This chapter describes some of the common emotional responses to infertility and its treatment. You may not experience everything described here, but some or much of it may be familiar. You and your partner will feel different things at different times and with varying degrees of intensity; there's no set rules about how people react. Having said that, there are certainly common experiences shared by everyone and a pattern to those experiences. Knowing that your feelings are completely normal and that other people have been there before can be a comfort. On the days when you feel like you're going crazy, it can help to know you're not the only one to have felt this way. Knowing what other people have experienced can also help you anticipate how you might feel in the future, and help you be a little more prepared.

Realistically, you will have very little opportunity to discuss the emotional implications of your treatment with your doctor—there just isn't time—but all clinics have counsellors available, and talking through some of these issues with them can really help. Specialist counsellors deal with these problems every day, and they have a broad understanding of much of what you might be going through. They can often provide a more thoughtful and considered response than well-intentioned but ill-informed friends and family. Some people find the one-on-one nature of a counselling session a little too much to start with, and prefer the less formal atmosphere of a support group; others prefer to share their feelings in the more private and anonymous environment of an Internet chat room.

If you are like most couples, however, you will probably end up sharing most of this with each other and a few select people—usually people with experience of infertility. Sometimes it can be difficult even to share your feelings with each other, and you might find yourselves mulling it all over in your head on your own. If you need to, talk to one of the clinic counsellors or, if they are not available, you can find out the name of a specialist infertility counsellor from the Australian and New Zealand Infertility Counsellors Association (see 'Information and resources').

> I was starting to become a little bit self conscious about the treatment, thinking, you know, you can't do this forever. People were probably quite sick of it I'm sure, friends and colleagues. I didn't want to become some obsessed neurotic woman who just never stopped. I wanted to remain terribly sensible and scientific about it all—if it wasn't going to work for me, then I'd just stop. Little did I know that was almost an impossible mental hurdle. It just wasn't that easy.
>
> Wendy

> We had both always very much wanted kids and finding out I had no sperm was a bit of a shock. Actually, it was devastating. My first reaction was that it is so unfair. I have three older brothers and they all have families and there has been no problem. I would have been happy to adopt right away, rather than do IVF, except that I really wanted Hannah to be pregnant—you know, to give birth and have that experience. But I never had a problem with adopting—or using donor sperm.
>
> Charles

Coping with infertility

Shock and disbelief

Probably the most common experience for couples when they initially discover they have a fertility problem is shock and disbelief. They might even think the test results are wrong or have been mixed up with someone else's. Most of us grow up with the expectation that, when the time and circumstances are right, we will find the right partner and have children. During adolescence we are constantly taught to be wary of our fertility, to abstain from sex, or to make sure we use contraception. Many of us spend our younger years desperately trying *not* to get pregnant, worrying that one forgotten pill, one act of unprotected sex, will result in an immediate pregnancy. We grow up believing conception is natural and easy and rarely do we question the fact that it will happen. It is not surprising, therefore, that we are shocked when it doesn't.

In general, people still tend to assume that infertility will lie with the woman, even though there is an equal chance of the problem being with either partner or with a combination of both. In some ways this makes it more difficult for the man if male factors are identified as the cause. Because many men genuinely do not expect the problem to lie with them, the shock and distress may be that much greater when they discover it does. Having children is a unique experience for both sexes, but the woman's capacity to carry the pregnancy, give birth and breastfeed means she has a more active role in the creation and nurturing of a child. When it comes to starting a family, the man has one important job—to provide sperm—and when something goes wrong with that, it can be devastating.

Men and women both define themselves through their genetic contribution to making a baby, but it is men's *only* biological contribution, and when they are unable to do this it is not unusual for them to feel an enormous sense of loss, disappointment, frustration or anger. Many men won't want to talk about it either, which may further reinforce their sense of isolation. Society still equates the capacity to father a child with masculinity, and in some cultures this belief is held very strongly. It is not uncommon for men who have problems with their sperm to struggle with issues of identity, masculinity and self-esteem. Many men experience strong feelings of guilt and some even feel that, in a way, they are failing to fulfil their marriage contract.

Similarly, much of female identity is tied up with carrying and giving birth to a child, and for many women being a mother is an important part of what it means to be a woman. Family expectations of women can be just as high and an inability to have a child can be perceived by others as failure. If female factor infertility is identified, the woman, too, may feel guilt at not being able to provide her partner with the child he wants. She may also experience feelings of inadequacy and low self-esteem. She has spent years dealing with periods and suffering through PMT, all with the expectation that one day her menstrual cycle will be put to good use. It is a huge shock and disappointment when that doesn't happen, and can seem very unfair.

A sense of loss

Once you get over the initial shock of a diagnosis, you can experience a profound sense of loss. It is this sense of loss, and the sadness and grief associated with it, that often underlies the whole experience of dealing with infertility and its treatment. The immediate loss is that of a much-wanted pregnancy, which would have resulted in a family, sons or daughters to love, nurture and share a life with, but there are other losses too. You may not get to provide grandchildren for your parents, or nieces or nephews for your siblings. You may not get to share the experience of motherhood with your own mother and sisters. So, too, men miss out on sharing the experience of fatherhood with their fathers and brothers. You may not get to pass on the family name or to continue the genetic line. You may not get to share this new stage of life with your friends who are all having babies. You may not get to plan things in the same way, and you may not get to move on. There are a hundred other ordinary things you miss out on: decorating the nursery, buying baby clothes, choosing a name, organising birthday parties, playing cricket on the beach, sharing your favourite children's books, deciding on schools, and much, much more.

It is not uncommon to feel angry or frustrated at this time, to feel cheated or robbed, to ask 'why me?' Many people experience feelings of resentment, shame, isolation, guilt and blame, and may even wonder about the purpose of their relationship if they are part of a couple. Infertility represents a huge loss of control too—so many things are taken out of your hands. All of a sudden, you are dependent on other people for something that was meant to be you and your partner's sole responsibility. Almost everybody expects they can make a baby and, even if you don't have much control over other aspects of your life, having children is something you can control. It can be hard to deal with the fact that this might not be so.

Even if the prognosis for having a baby with some form of treatment is good, it is still common to feel a sense of loss. You don't get to conceive in the privacy and intimacy of your own home, and your child won't be conceived as a result of a loving act—having a doctor insert an embryo into your uterus with a catheter on a cold Tuesday morning in his surgery is not quite the same. Everything to do with having a baby becomes very clinical, very quickly. You lose the possibility of spontaneous conception, of getting pregnant unexpectedly. You lose the excitement of doing a pregnancy test and the joy of the surprise. Rarely do you get to enjoy those first few weeks when only the two of you know, or have the pleasure of planning who and how you are going to tell. Quite simply, you will not conceive in the way you have always expected, in the way so many others seem to do with ease.

For many couples, however, the process of confronting their infertility and dealing with treatment can have a positive effect on their relationship. They might talk to each other more than they have done in the past, they might care for and nurture each other more and, as a consequence, their relationship may develop in new and different ways. It can bring them closer together. Many couples have also found that these positives can spill over into their lives as parents.

Reviving hope

Gradually, most people get over the initial shock and disappointment and begin to think about what treatment can offer. You acknowledge the fact that you have a medical problem, and accept that if you still want to create a family, you will have to do so with medical intervention. You might start to talk about the problem with a few close friends or family, and to think about who you will be able to seek support from in the future. The disappointment of the initial diagnosis slowly gives way to a renewed sense of optimism—there is a feeling there may be some answers out there after all. You can start to anticipate a pregnancy again and imagine having a child. Many people feel like they have taken back some control of their situation; that they are, at last, doing something useful and constructive. Although anxieties are experienced in the early days, starting treatment can be a positive time. You may not conceive your baby in the way you anticipated, and the path to having that baby might be a difficult one, but none of this really matters if, in the end, you are able to have a child.

If you are successful on your first or second cycle, as some people are, having a child will more than likely ensure these losses do not have a significant or lasting effect on you. You will be relieved, delighted and excited, and thankful that treatment is over, if only for now. You can get your life back on track and reactivate all the plans you'd put on hold.

If you are not successful to begin with you will find yourself doing repeated cycles. Almost all people who begin treatment do more than one stimulated cycle, and quite commonly they will do three or four. Some will do up to eight or ten cycles and a few will go beyond that. Because of the physical and emotional demands—and the financial costs—people often spread their cycles over an extended period of time. You may choose to do as many as four or five in a year, or may prefer to—or only be able to—do one or two. You might find you start with a rush of enthusiasm and do a few cycles back to back, and then slow down as time goes by. If you live a long way from a clinic, you may not be able to have treatment as often as you wish because of the additional expense and logistical problems of being treated some distance from home.

> My main coping mechanism involved glassware. Yup, I broke a lot of glassware. Had a few drinks—a bottle of gin and a packet of Alpines—and I broke a few glasses. But, seriously, one of my best coping mechanisms—and I would recommend it to everyone (other than having people to talk to about it) was exercise. I kept up the exercise the whole way through treatment and it was the only thing that enabled me to keep even a tenuous hold on my sanity. It gives you something else to focus on. Also, because the treatment does muck you around physically—the hormones . . . they make you fat, they make you tired, they make you hot and sweaty, you know, all those things—it does help if you feel physically fit. If you're feeling fat and tired and hot and sweaty at least you can feel well. I'm doing everything I can to not just end up like a blob.
>
> Andrea

Physical demands

The effects of IVF treatment are cumulative, for both the man and woman, but the physical demands are far greater on the woman. If you conceive relatively quickly, you should be fine—you'll deal with the pain and discomfort, and your optimism and the feeling that you are finally doing something positive will help you through the first couple of cycles. However, the physical demands become greater over time; the drugs and hormone injections, the general anaesthetics and medical procedures, the pain and discomfort, all take their toll. With repeated cycles, it is not unusual for the woman to feel physically exhausted, to feel weary on a daily basis, to feel overwhelmed. Where you were once fit and healthy and had lots of energy, you might now feel tired and sluggish most of the time. Where you went for a run or played sport, you now read a book or watch TV. Exercise becomes difficult and you might find yourself putting on weight with each cycle, weight that you can't get rid of before the next.

If you do a series of stimulated cycles over a number of months you can begin to forget how you used to feel when you weren't on treatment. I remember waking up one morning—a week or two after a treatment cycle had finished—and being surprised to find I actually had a bit of energy. I felt like I could face the day with some enthusiasm and could even manage a brisk walk to the shops. I felt like my old self again. It's almost as if you get so used to having the injections and procedures, and used to your body feeling completely out of sorts, that you find it difficult to remember how you once felt.

This is all completely normal, and the key to coping with it is to acknowledge that it happens to everybody. Having breaks between cycles can help you manage it because this allows your body time to recover, but also because it gives you a chance to remember what it's like not to be on IVF. A lot of energy goes into keeping yourself together emotionally and physically while you are actually having the treatment, and you need to give yourself time to rest and recuperate in between. Do nice things for your body: take a long bath, have a massage, go to the pool, do some gentle exercise. The constant assault on the body from IVF treatment is very difficult to sustain. Don't push yourself. Rest where you can, sleep when you need to, and take things as easy as your work and other responsibilities allow.

Many people find the few days leading up to their period, and the actual arrival of their period, a very difficult time. Not only are your hormones fluctuating so that you might feel teary or irritable anyway, but you have to deal with the confirmation that, once again, you are not pregnant. Getting your period is a very physical and unmistakeable reminder of your infertility, and it can leave you feeling down, angry or despondent. It is always the woman, too, who after getting her period, is the bearer of bad news to her husband or partner.

Men will experience this sense of loss too and many may also experience a sense of frustration and anguish watching their partners go through all this and not being able to fix it. Some also feel a sense of guilt if their partner is having to go through significant medical intervention when the problem doesn't actually lie with her.

A 30th birthday of a close friend was coming up and I just wanted to be able to let loose and relax, to have a drink. I also wanted to take a break while I still had embryos so when I went back I was going back to something easy, to a transfer.

Wendy

Each month I went through a cycle of optimism and hope, the trying, the disappointment and despair, and then trying again. It is just so cyclical, those emotions. It was a very difficult emotional time.

Darcy

I was failing at something that was very public, very normal, very easy to achieve . . . and I don't fail. It is very hard to be a failure at something that everybody else seems to be able to do very easily.

Lee

People say, 'How are you going? You seem to cope so well and you seem so calm.' And I'll say, 'Yeah, but you don't see me at home with Charles. I have my days.' But at the same time, I've also seen that being down about it, or blaming everyone else, doesn't get you anywhere.

Hannah

By the sixth failed cycle I was bitter and twisted. I'd see pregnant women in the supermarket and want to push my trolley into them—truly!

Andrea

You can't allow yourself to become numb to the whole thing, and I think that's the tough part. There's no way to step away from it and nobody, unless they are actually going through it, can relate.

Andrew

It was the to-ing and fro-ing trying to get pregnant that weighed as heavily on the mind [as the miscarriages], the times in between—tracking the cycle, ovulating, the obligation, and then two weeks later, the disappointment if it didn't work. That rhythm was controlling our lives, heaven and hell, heaven and hell. And there weren't many people who really saw that, they couldn't quite understand it. Some people said to me, 'Half the fun is trying,' but I didn't find it fun at all. I found it crushing. Or they said, 'Oh you lucky bugger,' or, 'Oh jeez, that's hard. You wanna beer?' And even women friends, I was surprised . . . they'd be sympathetic about a miscarriage, something tangible, but that was it.

Mark

Emotional ups and downs

The emotional consequences of treatment do not get any easier with time. A failed cycle brings disappointment, a second brings more, a third, fourth or fifth can bring frustration and anger, doubt and anxiety, and even despair. Each month you go through the not knowing, the hope and expectation of a pregnancy, and then the sadness and disappointment of a negative result. Even within one cycle there are so many emotional highs and lows: the drugs might stimulate your follicles really well and you produce ten great eggs, or they don't really do their thing and you end up with just one or two. They might fertilise and grow into healthy embryos, or fragment and die. Your transfer might be smooth and easy, or painful and difficult. You might conceive, but then miscarry. Hope and disappointment. Excitement and despair. Up and down. Up and down. This is the roller-coaster of emotion so commonly experienced by people on IVF.

It is important not to forget that—for the woman—this happens at a time when your hormones are all over the place. Your moods may be fluctuating wildly, and at different times you will probably feel tearful, depressed, angry, anxious or just plain fed up. This only compounds the difficulties of dealing with your treatment. It is tough for your partner too. He is living with you and going through all the ups and downs in his own way. He is on his own, separate roller-coaster. He may be coping with much of it alone, and not really talking to anyone else about how he feels. He may not know the best way to help you.

All this is heaped on to a continual and huge sense of loss that both of you are struggling with every day. It's not surprising you don't feel great—it is a very difficult time for the two of you and for your relationship. You may find you even stop talking to each other. Nurturing yourselves and the relationship by doing things together is really important—have a bath together, go to the movies, share a massage, take a sickie together.

I really tried to keep up my yoga, even though that was sometimes difficult in the second half of the cycle, after I'd had the transfer. But that was the most consistent thing for me, the yoga and my women's meditation group. I didn't really talk with them about the IVF but it was just good being with other women. Also, I did talk to other women who'd been on a program and that was really helpful. I'd certainly recommend anyone who goes on the program to work part-time if they can. And an understanding employer really helps as well.

Tracy

Loss of control

You may also feel that you have no control over what is happening to your life, and may experience that loss of control you felt at the very beginning of this process when you were first diagnosed. When you start a stimulated treatment cycle you are pretty much committed to a particular course of action for the next four to six weeks. Your day-to-day life is governed by your menstrual cycle and the various drugs used to manipulate it. Every time something comes up—a social function, a family gathering, a work do or sports fixture—you have to check the calendar and make an assessment of whether or not you'll be up to it: Will you be due for your egg pick-up? Will you be swollen and sore? Will you be exhausted or hormonal? Will it be around the date your period is due?

Important decisions that affect you both are made by doctors, nurses and administrators. It can seem as if you really have no say over what is happening to you and—for the woman—no control over what is happening to your body. IVF has a habit of taking over, and you may end up feeling that *it's* in charge, not you.

One of the things you can do to take back some control is to make sure you are both well informed about your condition and your treatment. You will feel more empowered if you are having input into the planning of your treatment. Read everything the clinic

> You do feel very powerless because you are being pushed from pillar to post. Knowing what to expect is helpful. Whether things are going well, or not so well, just knowing ahead of time exactly what's going on makes you far more able to cope with the situation.
>
> Wendy

> After the cycle with my egg donor didn't work I was very emotional. Up to that point I had been in control all the way. The biggest thing that started to dawn on me was that I'd been in control my whole life. I'd been successful at school. I'd been successful at sports. I'd been successful in my working life. I had a good career. My marriage was successful. So everything had been in my control. I was good at the things I did . . . but I couldn't do this basic thing of having a child.
>
> Tanya

provides, talk to other patients and research any specific conditions you have. Some people think this is obsessive or indulgent, but it's not; you can only benefit from educating yourself. The more you know, the more able you are to ask questions, and to participate actively in your treatment. You will feel more empowered if you are proactive about making appointments, quizzing your doctor and sharing in the decision making about your treatment. You can plan your treatment. You can decide when you want to take break.

> I guess what hit us through the whole course of treatment is how much it affects your life. Like for us, we had been wanting to go overseas to see Charles' family for three years and it was always, what if we're pregnant, you know, could I fly? There were so many holidays we didn't go on, so much we didn't do. You put your whole life on hold. It's only this last year that we've said, we're booking holidays, we're going whatever and, luckily, it has fit in pretty well.
>
> Hannah

Feeling stuck

As well as the problems you experience on a day-to-day basis, treatment will start to affect the bigger picture of your life. Your social

It was funny, all the IVF books say the husband should plan stuff, you know, nice things together, or distractions. But I had a really hard time planning anything, because I was always thinking when are we going to have this cycle? When are things going to happen? What if we did get pregnant? What if it doesn't work?

Charles

One of the hardest times for us was at the beginning of this year. During February and March we found out 15 people were pregnant, close friends and family. It was just everyone we bumped into . . . like an old boyfriend at the shops . . . 'What's new with you guys?' 'Oh not much. How about you?' 'Oh Tracey's 23 weeks pregnant.' 'Oh congratulations.' It's just like everyone throughout that time was pregnant.

Hannah

life may be curtailed because you're both exhausted, and you may not want to hang out with your usual crowd anyway if they all seem to be moving on without you. Holidays might be cancelled because the timing isn't right, renovations will be scaled down because of money, and career advancement will be put on hold. It may seem like you don't get much say about anything any more because everything has to be deferred to IVF. After a year or two of treatment, many people feel stuck—especially when friends and family have their first, then their second child. Even normal things—buying a new car, taking an overseas trip, getting a promotion—can make you feel like you're being left behind; another reminder of how your life is not moving on.

Where you can, try to include other things in your life, try to hang on to some of your other life goals and aspirations. This is difficult because treatment is so all-encompassing and doesn't leave you much time, energy or money for much else, but you may be able to set small, achievable goals—both individually and together. This will give you a sense that you are moving forward, at least in one part of your life. If you can manage it, taking a break can certainly help you to focus on a different aspect of your life for a change. Finding a different social circle—through a club, sport, or evening class—where people are not focused on babies, can also help.

> Trying to get pregnant and the miscarriages ruled our lives. It was just a grief that never went away because for the two weeks on, you're trying to conceive, then two weeks later you're dealing with the disappointment or the fear or the maybe. It was a really hard pattern and I found it almost impossible at times. The grief made any lovemaking . . . well it just didn't happen that often. It was like there was no space or emotional energy.
>
> Mark

Sex and intimacy

One of the most common effects of infertility and its treatment is a problem with sex and intimacy. It is not uncommon for couples to have sex very infrequently throughout the time they are having treatment, or for sex to become a bit mechanical. Some couples stop having sex altogether. In the first place, you may have been having sex at specific times to coincide with ovulation, which has likely taken some of the fun and spontaneity out of it. The man, especially, may feel pressured to perform, and feel as though he is no more than some kind of stud, wanted only for his sperm. Problems with maintaining an erection are also not uncommon. You might both just be a bit more weary than usual, especially the woman who will be tired and under par from the effects of medication and treatment. The hormones may also have a negative effect on her libido. What was once an intimate and personal act has now become all rather clinical—there is really nothing very sexy about IVF.

On top of all this there are some bigger issues. Sex may have been about pleasure in the past, but it is now about conception. For many couples, sex during IVF just reminds them of what is not happening—of the fact that they are not getting pregnant. It can reinforce your sense of loss and can actually be quite a sad thing. Understandably, many people choose to avoid it. If you've been having treatment for a while and have had a number of disappointments, you will be grieving, and might well have underlying feelings of sadness much of the time. No one feels like sex in these circumstances.

Even after treatment is over—whether you have a child or not—there can be a time where you re-think what sex is about. Your sex life may return easily to your pre-IVF days, but don't be surprised if it requires a little readjustment. The role of sex in your relationship—and each partner's expectations about it—may have to be redefined. If you have a problem, or are worried, talk to each other, or talk to a counsellor. There are a lot of ways to be physically intimate and enjoy each other sexually. This might be a time to try something new and different—use your imagination or look at one of the many books on the subject.

> One of the disservices I did Mark is that I asked him not to talk to anyone about it [our difficulty having a baby]. I felt so aware that it was my failure and I didn't give Mark space to talk about it. I made my own decisions about who I talked to about it, and how much I shared. So I was doing that, but I hadn't given Mark permission to do that.
>
> Lee

Stress on relationships

Problems with sex can put a strain on a relationship—or a strain on the relationship can cause problems with sex. You are both dealing with some enormously difficult, personal and complex issues. Your self-esteem might have taken a battering and you

The biggest issue I had was, because I work from home and run my own business, I don't actually have a lot of the contact most people who go into a workplace have. So it was actually a lot more insular from my point of view. I was sort of having to cope with it on my own and didn't get to discuss it very much, which was hard. We were both one another's support network to a great extent and sometimes it was hard to prop one another up, especially if you're feeling flat—you're trying to prop the other one up, not the best situation to be in but you've got to do it.

Andrew

I've often said it's incredible how different people respond to IVF in different ways. IVF in itself is enough to drive wedges—significant wedges—into a relationship. I was sort of thinking, 'Look, if our relationship can survive this, if we can stick together—we can survive any damn thing.'

Andrew

By the fifth cycle our emotions were just . . . Well, put it this way, I think we were ready to have a break. We were fighting and things were pretty stressful. It runs both your lives, the program, and it was starting to consume me. There just wasn't much joy happening in our lives. The treatment was taking over.

Tracy

At the start we were very together—we were going through the whole process together—but by the end . . . IVF is lonely, the loneliest thing I've ever done, even though you're with your partner. I think I felt even more alone towards the end. We were going through different emotions. Greg was probably beginning to question whether it would ever happen and I was fearful about whether he would want to keep trying.

Tracy

> As a bloke I didn't feel left out, but sometimes it was like I was just along for the ride. I'd just give the needle and that was it. I guess we're a bit like a sperm bank anyway—you do what you do and then nine months later . . . But I tried to get involved as much as I could. I couldn't feel sick for Tracy which I wanted to sometimes, but I tried to be there as much as I could and, like with the needles, make sure I could actually do it. It saved us a lot of time but it was also one part that I could do. All the emotional stuff and the body changes and everything that Tracy had to go through was pretty hard, and I felt sorry for her having to go through all this and then get a negative result.
>
> Greg

might be re-examining the part you play in this relationship. You are both being subjected to all sorts of intimate questioning and invasive tests and procedures. The woman, especially, may be worn down by ongoing treatment. Where you might have previously made up pretty quickly after a fight, you might find some ill-feeling spilling over to the next day.

Your social life has probably taken a dive and you might have no money to splash out on a weekend away or a dinner out. You might disagree about your next course of treatment, about when and what to do, or how long you want to continue trying. There might be additional pressures from members of your family which aren't helping either. All of these things are difficult to handle, and they can place a strain on your relationship.

It takes an enormous amount of energy just to survive ongoing IVF treatment, and it should come as no surprise if you are a little more irritable than usual, if you have less patience, or if you sometimes end up taking out your frustrations on each other. You might find yourselves bickering more than you used to and you won't be the only ones to have the occasional full-on row. Some people close down completely, withdrawing from their partners as a way of coping, and end up feeling distant and alone.

It's a tough time and you may need to remind yourselves that you're on the same team—you might want to do something fun together, to remember what you love about each other. Certainly, for many couples, the struggles of IVF have brought them closer together; more than ever before they have had to share their emotions, to love, nurture and support each other. This can have a lasting positive effect on a relationship—if you can get through IVF, you can get through anything. Whatever your situation, the key to maintaining the health of your relationship is good, open communication.

At the time [of the recurrent miscarriages], we probably didn't talk about it a lot. I probably talked to Mark more about my needs than listened to Mark about his needs. I don't think there was as much space for him to talk about how it was for him. And he was really looking after me and making sure I was okay. I was also taking care of him by not telling him stuff because I didn't want to worry him or burden him further. Mark spent more time at work and more time working on the house, and buried himself into a whole lot of other stuff.

Lee

We have very different ways of coping. My husband closes up. He doesn't talk about it. We both retreat to our own little boxes.

Tanya

Every once in a while Hannah's friends ask how she's going, but nobody ever asks me. There was one time, a couple of friends actually asked me about it, but it is very rare that anyone actually asks the guy. I mostly just talked to Hannah.

Charles

> The whole thing builds up after a time and when you're feeling flat, trying to buoy your partner up is not the easiest thing in the world. But it's sort of really tough, I guess, when you're in a position where there's a failed cycle and you feel . . . well regardless of how you feel, you've actually got to support your partner.
>
> Andrew

> I had good and bad responses from people. The bad responses were when people were insensitive or when they just didn't really respond at all, people who didn't get in touch with me again, or who gave a one-word response like, 'Gee', or, 'that's bad luck'. I think all I wanted from anybody was, 'I'm sorry' . . . just for them to register. Maybe they didn't care about children, but it was a blow to me. Good responses were where people said, 'I don't know what you're going through, I don't pretend to know, but it's pretty big stuff.' Probably the easiest people to talk to were the ones who had experienced this in the same way, the cycle of wanting children and not being able to, but they were few and far between.
>
> Mark

Communication

There might never have been a time in your relationship where talking to each other openly and honestly was more important. Often communication breaks down because the pain of what of you are both going through is just too much, and it's easier to withdraw into yourselves rather than have to deal with somebody else. Often, ironically, communication problems arise from a desire to protect each other. You may both be aware of how much the other is hurting and not want to add to their burden by expressing your own fears, doubts or sadness. Sometimes people don't express what they feel because they are worried their partner may use the fact that they

> I suppose my main way of coping was that I threw myself into work. I have a cushy and thoroughly boring job, which has never been a big part of my life, and it was an even greater irrelevance in the face of the really important stuff that was happening to me. I moved into another area and it was a full-on, seven-day a week thing. I relished it because I could no longer deal with Lee's grief. I was just full up with grief after the third miscarriage, and Lee was just so sad in a way she had never been. I couldn't help her. I couldn't fix the problem. And I threw myself into the work which is something I had never done before. It was an escape. There was a new bunch of people there and if I went out I went out with them on big drinking nights. I sort of kept that up for about eight months. I still had the house to work on, physical jobs, any project that I could absorb myself in. I would have bought six cars to work on as a distraction if that had been possible.
>
> Mark

are struggling as a reason to stop treatment when they really don't want to. If you do not share your feelings there can be a tendency to drift apart, especially if, on top of this, you aren't being sexual or physically intimate.

The other problem that often arises is that men and women deal with things differently. It's not the same for everyone, of course, but it is not uncommon for men to deal with their feelings by doing something practical: going for a jog, fixing the car, painting the deck, playing sport, or mowing the lawn. They keep themselves busy, and try to remain positive by not dwelling on the problem too much. After all, what's the point in talking about it? Their partner, on the other hand, might want to do exactly that. For her, talking about it may be the best thing she can do. She may want to express her feelings, to share these with him, and want him to express his feelings in return.

His coping mechanisms might be perceived by her as indifference, or a lack of care, or even abandonment. Her desire to talk might make him feel overwhelmed, pushing him even further away. Getting through this involves understanding and acceptance of the different coping strategies you both employ. One way of dealing with this is to set aside some time—maybe an hour a week—to talk about what is happening. She gets to talk about her feelings, to cry or feel sad, and he listens and, if he wants to, talks a little about how he feels. In return, she tries to understand that he's not uncaring or abandoning her, and doesn't hassle him the next day when he disappears into the shed for a few hours. However you decide to do it, the important thing is that you keep talking, even if that seems a really hard thing to do. Reading a book together—like this one—can also help.

> We kept having breaks between cycles and at the time we thought we were doing the best thing, but looking back we wished we'd just kept going. Obviously, it's hard doing a cycle and you think, 'Okay, let's take a break, we'll take a month or two off and do another one.' But thinking about it now, it would have been a much better idea to do a few cycles in a row, and then maybe take a couple of months off and do a few more in a row, because you look back and you think of all the time you wasted. If we had done more cycles we might have had a different result, or we might have known things earlier. But then if we hadn't had those breaks maybe now we would be looking back and saying, 'We should have had more breaks!' It's kind of frustrating.
>
> Charles

The will to keep going

Everything described above is a normal response to what you are going through, and pretty much everyone experiences these things to some degree. Dealing with infertility is largely a matter of managing these feelings on a day-to-day basis and doing whatever works for you. Many people successfully navigate this difficult path

I got onto the Internet and I typed in the name of this protocol my specialist had recommended. I was trying to find people I could talk to and this site popped up and it was a bulletin board where I could talk to other people on IVF. They were other Melbourne girls, people who were seeing my doctor. It was like this whole world, it was like group therapy every day, all afternoon. When I was supposed to be working, I was chatting to these people. It was very positive. Suddenly I didn't feel anything like alone. For example, we'd go out for dinner and some fool would make a comment that normally would have just sent me hiding into my shell because I couldn't bear to deal with it. I could log on to this site and say, 'I just had dinner and this idiot said blah, blah . . . ' and then everyone would come on and say, 'Oh yeah, that happened to me . . . don't you hate it?' and, 'Oh my God, how do you feel?' And it was so good to have that outlet, to be able to vent. It made a huge difference.

Andrea

The fourth cycle was devastating for me. It's the odds, you know, you have a 25 per cent chance so you think it's going to have to be this one. Everyone had built our hopes up. Tracy's meditation group had some visualisation thing, and it was all going to happen. That all got a bit much actually, when people would say, 'I can just feel it's going to happen. 'It's a full moon', or whatever. I always felt more like, well the transfer done, let's forget about it for two weeks and then we'll know either way.

Greg

I started seeing a counsellor, one that came free at work. That probably wasn't the best, but it was great to have someone who was there to listen and to throw things back at me. I'd never thought I'd ever have to see a counsellor. I never wanted to, but by that time I put my hand up and said, 'Yes, please.'

Mark

and after, say, three or four treatments, have a successful pregnancy and move on with their lives. The situation begins to change—it gets more difficult—if you have repeated treatments that do not result in a successful pregnancy, or if you have repeated miscarriages. This is when things can get really tough.

You will almost certainly find that your treatment gets more difficult to manage the more cycles you do. Familiarity helps and can relieve some anxieties but, in almost all cases, the longer you undertake treatment the more difficult it gets. There are lots of reasons for this. The treatment has a huge impact on both of you emotionally, and on the woman physically, and this tends to be cumulative. Treatment affects your relationships, your work and your day-to-day lives, and can become completely overwhelming. After a while, you might begin to fear that it may never work. You might lose faith in doctors and medical science. You may no longer expect to find answers that in the beginning you thought would be forthcoming. You might lose all hope. You might struggle to keep things in perspective. You might find that time just runs out. If you do end up on the IVF treadmill, you will inevitably find yourselves dealing with ongoing feelings of sadness and grief.

> I was approaching 40 and in therapy, talking about my grief at the possibility of not having a child and trying to entertain the thought of being childless. This was extremely difficult. I struggled with finding the meaning of my life, the purpose of my life. But hope is very seductive and it enticed me to the next step time and time again.
>
> Darcy

Sadness and grief

Infertility is about loss, and loss is what causes us to grieve. We normally associate grief with someone dying, but people going

I have a distinct memory of being so certain that it [getting pregnant] would happen and having this genuine shock the second and third time it didn't happen. I never thought it would be the first time, but I was shocked when it didn't happen the second time.

Wendy

I just kept referring back to all those statistics that I was constantly told were on my side. I was under 30, there was nothing really wrong, blah, blah. It was almost a negative thing having all those statistics on my side.

Wendy

I think when I had the first miscarriage I was about eight weeks, the second, seven weeks, and the third and fourth about five and four weeks. There wasn't—there isn't—a lot of space to grieve because having a miscarriage is defined as normal. It's sort of like, 'Oh well. It's just a miscarriage. It happens all the time, and it's normal. You'll be fine.' But it wasn't fine. It was really sad. There just isn't much space to grieve. They are not babies. No one defines them as babies, but they are babies, it's just that they are so small. It is still a loss and there isn't much space to talk about it.

Lee

through infertility often experience a sense of grief too. There are so many things you thought you'd have, so many expectations that won't be fulfilled, so much love to give and receive that now has nowhere to go. Each unsuccessful cycle involves an embryo—a potential life, a possible son or daughter—that is lost to you forever. That's a very sad thing, especially if you've said goodbye to lots of embryos over months or years. If you've experienced an ectopic pregnancy or a miscarriage, this feeling might be worse, especially if it's happened more than once.

I had another transfer and we were really hopeful. It was absolutely perfect: an easy transfer and a really good embryo. I was really hopeful. I got the phone call from the clinic at work—I should never have been in the office. I just fell to bits that time. I don't know why that was different to the previous times, but I fell to bits. I didn't cope at all. I ended up having to take two days off work. That's when I started to realise, when it started to hit me. I think the first and second unsuccessful tries were okay, but the third time it was starting to hit home that this might not happen.

Tanya

People don't know what to say. Everyone is very supportive in those first two weeks after you've had the transfer. You know, 'You can do it. You can do it. Up that hill.' But people don't know what to say to you when you've had a negative result, so they don't say anything. You feel uncomfortable for them as well. And then, over time, it gets even more difficult, because it's another cycle they've been there to build you up through, and another negative result.

Tracy

I was subsumed by caring, worrying and witnessing how distraught, how terribly defeating it [a second miscarriage] was for Lee. The grief was immense and I never dreamed it would be like that. So I was just trying really hard to support Lee. It was secondary what I felt. Lee was the one who was pregnant.

Mark

When you start treatment you tend to be quite optimistic, which is a completely reasonable and normal response as many people achieve a positive outcome after a few cycles. It is always important to be hopeful. But over time, if treatment is repeatedly unsuccessful, this can become more and more difficult. You might ask yourself what chance do you have of getting pregnant this time, when you didn't get pregnant the last five times. The effect of all those negative results, all those lost embryos, builds up over time and becomes very difficult to manage. If you have experienced repeated negative pregnancy tests or recurrent miscarriages, you are effectively suffering from chronic loss and you need to give yourself a chance to grieve. Allowing yourself to grieve means naming what you are going through as a loss—even if other people really don't see it that way—and giving yourselves permission to feel sad about it. It means expressing that sadness in whatever way is appropriate for you—crying, going for a long walk, feeling down, taking time off work. You don't have to keep it all bottled up. You don't have to cope all the time. You are allowed to say, 'I feel awful. This is really sad.'

Everyone experiences grief differently, but there are commonalities in that experience. For some it may last a short time, and for others it may extend over months or even years. It may come in sudden waves or bursts, or it may be a constant underlying feeling that never really goes away. The process of grieving begins with acknowledging your loss and believing in the reality of your situation. It means knowing that, despite all your efforts, the likelihood of your conceiving a child now is slim. It means allowing yourself to experience how painful that is. Once you have started to accept you might never have the family you always wanted, you might feel angry—even if you are not normally an angry person. 'Why me?' you might well ask. What have I done to deserve this? You might look around and see all sorts of people who you think are less deserving of having children than you. For a while—for a long time even—you might find it difficult to be happy for other people who are getting pregnant or having babies.

You will probably go through a period of mourning where you feel sad for yourself and your partner, and for your loss. You will regret that things turned out this way and wish they were different. You may even apportion blame—something you or your partner did, either recently or in the past. You may be doubtful of your ability to control other aspects of your life, or other things that may happen to you. You may feel scared or lack confidence. You might feel more and less sane on different days. You might really struggle to see anything hopeful or bright in the future. You might feel that if you can't have children nothing really matters any more.

One of the difficulties faced by people experiencing the chronic loss of infertility is that the loss is often not recognised by other people in our lives; it certainly isn't recognised by society in general. Normally, a death or significant loss is associated with appropriate rituals that help us acknowledge it, mourn for it, and begin to move on. Certain feelings and types of behaviour are accepted, even expected: tears, sadness, pain, emptiness, a loss of hope. Most people who go through infertility experience all these feelings to some degree, but are often not able to express them, or to share them, and are often not supported in getting through them. The usual condolences and support that people offer—writing a card, sending flowers, cooking a meal, just being a shoulder to cry on—don't always happen. The grief of infertility can be very isolating.

One way of dealing with the sense of loss is to create your own rituals—your own way of saying goodbye to all the embryos, the miscarriages, the children you never had. Some people plant a flower or a tree in their garden, or put a bench or chair on the porch. Some people find a special place, by a river or in a park, where they go to grieve quietly. Some people say a prayer, or light a candle, or read a poem or write a letter. Some people pick a day in the year where they do something special to honour and remember their loss. It's a way of respecting the life that you lost or never had, a way of restoring dignity to the experience you've been through. It's not morbid or gloomy, but a helpful way for you and your partner to move forward.

For most people the sense of loss remains; it's not something you get over or that goes away, but its impact on your life is reduced. Over time, you will be able to redirect the emotional energy that's going into grieving into other more positive areas of your life. Gradually, you will feel less sad and more hopeful, and your life will begin to take shape again.

> I was an absolute mess [after a negative pregnancy test]. For three days I just cried and cried and cried. My husband was shocked. He didn't know what to do. He'd never seen me like this and he'd known me for a long time. He just couldn't believe it. I think that's when we needed support. But at the time I don't think I realised any of that. I didn't recognise it.
>
> Tanya

> After the third failed cycle our optimism was waning a bit. I probably got pretty depressed, but I maybe got more depressed for Tracy because I could see how devastated she was. I was the same I suppose, I just probably didn't show it as much.
>
> Greg

Depression

A sense of sadness, of feeling down, is a normal response to infertility and ongoing failed treatment. This doesn't mean, however, that you have to suffer through it on your own or that you can't get help. Talking to each other is good, but sometimes that might just be too difficult. If you are both feeling particularly down it can be useful to talk to someone outside the relationship—friends, family, a support group or an infertility counsellor. It is not uncommon for people who have been having treatment for a long time to suffer from mild depression, which in some cases can become more severe.

You may find that the coping mechanisms you have been using to help you get through just don't seem to be working any more. Where you used to bounce back after each treatment cycle, now you don't. Maybe you've started to lose hope. Maybe your relationship is really starting to suffer.

Lots of people going through treatment experience periods of depression, and it's actually quite normal. It is not uncommon to experience any or all of the following: not wanting to get up in the morning, crying a lot or unexpectedly, feeling sad or withdrawn, not wanting to talk to people, feeling short-tempered or impatient, losing interest in things you used to enjoy, feeling tired and apathetic, having no energy or enthusiasm for anything, being unable to cope at work, having difficulty sleeping, feeling negative or without hope, feeling angry, vulnerable or despairing.

Problems really only arise if these feeling don't go away—if they persist over a number of weeks—or if they start to have a serious or prolonged negative impact on your life. If you feel you are slipping into a depression, it is really important you don't try to cope alone and you seek professional help. One of the problems with this sort of clinical depression is that often the person going through it doesn't actually realise until someone—usually a counsellor—tells them. Often they can only see it when they look back later. A counsellor can help you to identify exactly what you are going through—whether it is a perfectly normal response to grief or something more—and suggest some strategies that might help you get through this difficult time.

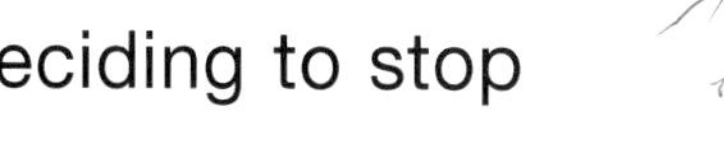

Deciding to stop

At some stage in this process—and it is different for everyone—you will start to face the possibility that treatment is not going to work for you. This is an especially difficult decision. In some instances

I was over 40 now, working through my grief, and looking for other meaning and purpose in my life. I felt a little bit more settled with not being a mother. Just. Enough to be able to say, 'I'll try a couple more times, but there has to be an ending. I have to let go'. Hope, as I said before, is very seductive. It is like a drug and it is very hard to give up.

Darcy

While you are still having treatment you haven't accepted the possibility that you'll never have children. I ask myself, is it that deep down I believe the treatment is going to work, or is it maybe more that I'm not prepared to accept the alternative? While I'm still doing treatment I'm not childless. I can't say that I don't believe it's going to work, because deep down I must. But for me the focus is more about, if I stop what does that say? What does that mean?

Wendy

I still can't imagine getting to the point where I have to accept that I won't have children, because surely there are other alternatives for treatment out there. But I did start to get very down this year when I realised I don't have that many choices. I am at the point now where I'm thinking, 'God, what's wrong with me?'

Wendy

you may discover something—the quality of your eggs is not good, or they're just not fertilising—that makes you reconsider your options. In other cases, your doctor will have no explanation for your failure to conceive despite many cycles of treatment. Where, at the beginning, you thought there would be answers and solutions, you now find there are none. There are still many things doctors

It was really important to stop trying to get pregnant [after recurrent miscarriages]. It was really important to give myself permission to stop. I know someone who had seven miscarriages, and I know someone who used heparin and aspirin and got pregnant. But I just think, I did what was best for me and everybody is different.

Lee

I decided to have a year off treatment. I didn't think about it for months and when I started to get to the end of that twelve-month period I was really uptight and I didn't understand why, but it was because I was going to have to make a decision [to try again to get pregnant or stop]. The twelve months came and went and I just put it off, and put it off, and thought, 'It's not the right time now', or, 'We're going to move house, let's not think about it'. Then, interestingly enough, about six weeks ago I discovered I was showing signs of menopause at 42, so the decision was made for me. That gave me closure.

Tanya

We have always had a timeline, because we didn't want to go through it for umpteen years. Before they changed the rules there had always been a six-cycle limit so I sort of had that in my head. You have to have a timeframe, for your sanity, because IVF's no life. You have to set time limits so you can move onto different things.

Charles

don't know. The reality is that IVF doesn't work for everyone, and it is such a chronically difficult journey, with so many disappointments, so many physical demands and so much emotional pain, that there is a limit to how long you can do it. That limit, of course, is different for everyone, and will depend on a number of factors.

There were certainly moments where I thought this isn't ever going to happen and I was terrified and that was sort of what kept me going. I could not bear the thought of facing a future without a family—I just couldn't bear it—so that's what kept me going. Every now and then I'd say, 'It's not going to work. We won't do it any more,' and then I'd say, 'But it might. I can't stop yet'.

Andrea

We got pregnant again—a fourth time—but that didn't last long at all. Even before that Lee was so defeated and so resigned that she wasn't going to be a mother . . . she said she couldn't do this any more which brought up all sorts of feelings for me. For her it meant stepping away from her life, our life, saying it's not going to happen, I'm not going to be a mother.

Mark

You might find the financial strain of ongoing treatment is just too much and you may start to resent spending money on IVF when it could be better spent on so many other things. You might be fed up with the restrictions it places on aspects of your life—your career and other interests. You might feel that to continue would jeopardise your relationship. You might just be, as many couples are, physically and emotionally exhausted—wrung out with nothing left. Gradually, for all or any of these reasons, there will come a time when you will *not* want to do a cycle more than you want to do one. If having children and undergoing treatment has been your exclusive focus for some time, giving up will be very difficult. If you have other important things in your life, other goals, other plans waiting to be put into place, it will help.

Deciding to stop is usually a process rather than a sudden decision, and you might start to think about the possibility of stopping long before you actually do. It can help to start laying the groundwork for future plans or introducing some new things into your life to shift the emphasis away from having a child. Some couples decide to take a long break and review the situation in, say, six or twelve months. This way they can move towards stopping without actually having to make a final decision. Some couples leave a final embryo in storage with a view to coming back to treatment later, but don't actually do so. Many couples finish treatment and go home quietly hoping that—even after everything they've been through—they might still conceive naturally. They put other plans in place, though, so if the miracle doesn't happen, they are still moving forward.

Sometimes a woman may find it extremely difficult to give up, even when the treatment is having an ongoing negative effect on her and her relationship, and even where doctors are suggesting her chances of conceiving are very slim. She simply cannot let go of the need to have a child. In this instance it can be useful to acknowledge that there will be a time in the future when you will stop having treatment, and to think about when that time will be. It doesn't have to be now or even in a year, but it will come eventually. If you assume you will not be having treatment much past the age of 45, and if you are, say, 38 now, ask yourself, do you have seven years of treatment in you? If not, maybe 42 is a more reasonable cut-off point, or even 40. Then you can think about how you are going to manage those four or two years. You can then develop a realistic plan in consultation with your doctor, but this plan has an end. In this way, you and your partner can start to look to the future, and think about how you are going to rebuild your lives.

Having a baby after infertility treatment

If you have a baby after a relatively short time of infertility and treatment, you may not experience any ongoing or long-term effects as a result. If, however, that baby comes after a long period of infertility and a lot of treatment, you may experience some difficulties

that you might not expect. The baby, of course, will be the answer to your dreams—the long hoped for outcome of years of trying. In many ways its arrival will bring relief and resolution, but it doesn't automatically wipe out everything you've been through. You still carry that history of loss with you; you still had to undergo all those years of invasive treatment and the huge emotional struggles that went with them. Those things just don't go away. Now, of course, with the baby, they may no longer be associated with sadness and loss to the same degree, but they are still part of your personal history, part of who you are now. You will always have gone through the experience of infertility. For most people that experience can be allocated a back-seat—at least for a while. It will be just something that sits quietly in the background with other parts of your personal history.

Some people who conceive after infertility may experience difficulties in the early days after their babies are born. The first few months of parenting are difficult for everyone—there are all sorts of new emotional and practical challenges to deal with, usually on little sleep. Everyone goes through a period of adjustment and, in differing degrees, may experience feelings of shock, inadequacy, fear, or just feel exhausted and overwhelmed. Once the baby is at home, they might find looking after it is tiring and more challenging than they thought—many people do. They will be relieved when the grandparents come over so they can catch up on a couple of hours' sleep, or have half an hour to themselves. All of this is completely normal.

If you have been trying to get pregnant for many years, it can be very difficult to admit to any of these feelings. When you have wanted this baby for so long—and everybody knows it—how can you be anything other than completely grateful all the time? How can you possibly suggest that having this baby is anything other than absolutely fantastic and that you are totally happy? Parents who conceive through infertility treatment sometimes find it more difficult to admit that things are difficult—even though that's completely normal—and may find it more difficult to ask for help. Some people won't want to admit those feeling to their partner; some will struggle to admit them to themselves. Other new parents can talk about these difficulties, complain and even joke about them, but IVF parents will not generally give themselves permission to do that.

If this is your experience, it's important that, at the very least, you talk to each other—it is quite likely you are both feeling the same way, and just discovering this can be a relief. It is entirely okay for you to feel fed-up some days, to feel like this wasn't quite what you expected, to want to hand your screaming bundle to your mother while you go for a walk around the block. Try not to hold yourself to an impossible standard, and try to keep feelings of guilt at bay. Again, if things get really tough, talk to an infertility counsellor who understands these issues. Just because you now have a baby, it doesn't mean that your infertility no longer has an impact.

Secondary infertility

Secondary infertility is where you are unable to conceive or carry a baby to term after you have already had one or more successful pregnancies. Most people presume that if they conceived reasonably easily the first time, they will conceive reasonably easily the second time too, and, while this is often the case, it is not always so. Sometimes this may just be a matter of perception—if, for example, it took you three months to get pregnant with your first child and you are not pregnant after, say, eight or ten tries the second time, you might think it is taking a long time, but in actual fact you were lucky the first time and are now just within the normal range. If you are still not pregnant after 12 to 18 months of trying, then there may be a problem. In some cases this may be identifiable—advanced age or a medical condition—but, as with primary infertility, the reason may remain a mystery.

People with secondary infertility may find their frustration and feelings of loss are not really understood. Because there are many people who don't have even one child, there is a sense you aren't really allowed to feel sad or disappointed that you can't have a second; that in wanting another you are somehow greedy or ungrateful. You may be on the receiving end of well-meant, but unhelpful comments like, 'at least you've got one', and, 'be grateful for what you have'. Having one child, however, may not lessen the pain of not being able to have another, of not providing a sibling for your son or daughter, of not having the family you always imagined you would. Many of the feelings described in this chapter can apply just as much to people suffering from secondary infertility.

Summing up

No two couples experience infertility in the same way, but if it is possible to draw some generalisations from the experience of going through treatment, they might look something like this:

- Treatment is emotionally demanding and at different times you may feel sad, angry, frustrated, depressed, anxious, elated or a whole range of other things. Many people talk about it being an 'emotional roller-coaster'—up one minute and down the next, month after month. It certainly can be.
- Managing the effects of infertility can place an enormous strain on your relationship—patience, understanding and good communication skills will help. If you can maintain your sense of humour and laugh occasionally, you will be able to stay with the treatment longer.
- Men and women will approach the problem differently and may develop very different ways of coping. Husbands and partners may at times feel awkward and unsure, insecure about their role, or just plain left out.
- IVF treatment is physically demanding, especially for the woman, who generally has to manage most of the hormones

and surgery. The drugs can have unpleasant side effects and procedures are often uncomfortable, sometimes painful.

- Having a well qualified and experienced doctor, with whom you feel safe and trust, is essential; having nurses and administrators who are sympathetic is a bonus.
- You will probably find that talking to others struggling with infertility—friends, a support group or a counsellor—will help. Reading or searching the Internet for information can also be useful.
- Some forms of treatment are very expensive and will likely be an enormous drain on your financial resources. Your lifestyle may change with the combined effect of treatment and having less money generally.
- You will have to balance the level of secrecy—who you do and don't tell—with your need for understanding and support. You may find that some friends and family do not handle your situation as well as you would like them to, but others will surprise you.
- If you are single, it can be especially tough, and you will need good friends and family members to support you. If you're in a lesbian relationship you may have additional difficulties to face, but you may also have two chances at conception.
- You will try to not let infertility and its treatment take over your life, but sometimes it will, despite your best efforts. If your treatment doesn't work it may bring enormous sadness; if it does you will feel all the effort has been worth it.

9

Moving forward

Life without children

If you conceive and carry a baby successfully, moving on with your life will be easy—pretty soon your focus will shift to the pregnancy and the birth, and your days ahead will be filled with the challenges and rewards of raising your family. If you don't end up with a baby it will be much less easy to bear but, sooner or later, you will have to start looking to the future and imagining what your life will look like without children. Making the transition to a life where you are not trying to conceive—where you don't have children and know you never will—takes time and is not easy. For a long while now your focus will have been on creating a family, something that—if it had eventuated—would have reshaped your lives significantly. But if it doesn't happen you are left with the life you always had and with what can feel like an enormous gap. How can you move forward? How can you fill that gap?

For many people, it can be extremely difficult to imagine ever feeling happy, contented or whole again, or to believe that anything positive can come out of this difficult time. Your infertility, your childlessness, won't go away, and the sadness it carries with it will probably always be with you. Though it might be impossible to imagine right now, there are other ways you can enjoy life and feel happy and whole again. As with any grief, it takes time to work through and everyone responds differently. You will have better and worse days, but slowly, as the months pass, the pain will ease and more positive feelings will replace it.

There are some good things about reaching this stage. Finishing treatment can be an enormous relief; after all this time you finally get some control back over your life. You can start to plan again, to reactivate things long put on hold—you don't have to scrutinise the calendar every time someone suggests doing something. You can go away for the weekend, decorate the house, buy some new clothes—you can spend money on something other than treatment. You can throw out all the drugs and needles lurking in the bathroom, and stop worrying about what your body is and isn't doing. You can forget about all the pills, injections and nasal sprays, all those speculums and catheters, those interminable blood tests and scans. You can start to renegotiate the role of sex in your life and maybe return to a time when it was about fun and pleasure not about procreation. You can start to make plans, to focus on your relationship, your work or other parts of your life. You can remember what it feels like to be you again. You can have your life back.

If you have stopped trying because of recurrent miscarriages, it can also be an enormous relief. It may have been a long time since conception was a wholly joyous thing for you because of the enormous fears that came with any pregnancy. Once you make the decision to stop, you no longer have to live with that fear, and you never have to go through another miscarriage.

Anniversaries and reminders

Once you stop trying you may find that certain days or particular events bring back painful memories that can trigger feelings of sadness and loss. These days or events are a reminder of how you

I was really starting to question what I was doing [trying to conceive after repeated miscarriages], my own sense of identity, my own sense of self-esteem, my own contribution to the world in which I lived. I felt like my world had shrunk. I joke about lying on the couch eating Chocolate Royals, but I was really sad. I felt stuck and out of control. I was existing in an increasingly and narrowly focused world, focused on me and my pain. I didn't feel any sense of the broader world. I felt like I needed to actually take a step back and put things in a bit of perspective.

Lee

I started to think maybe this isn't going to happen, and what do I do if it doesn't happen, and who am I? Who will I be if I am not a mother? If I'm not able to enjoy that with Mark? And that's when I started to have this sort of alternative plan, that maybe I needed to go off and do something different.

Lee

We discussed the whole infertility issue and I always said it has to do with outcomes. Now, worst-case scenario, we don't have a child and we have a pretty good life, so you're either positive or status quo. Whereas the worst-case scenario on the other hand [having testicular cancer] was terminal or reduced quality of life, so for me it wasn't that difficult.

Andrew

stayed in the same place while others moved on, a reminder of what you haven't been able to share with your partner and family. Holidays can be especially difficult—Christmas, Easter, the summer—the times when kids are off school and families are enjoying themselves. A spring fete at your local school, a carols by candlelight concert, a community fun day, even a toy sale at a department store can be difficult. Mother's Day and Father's Day are tough, and birthdays can just be a reminder of the lasts ticks of your biological clock. Lots of people have their own personal anniversaries: a positive pregnancy test, a miscarriage or ectopic pregnancy, the date of the first or last cycle. The birth of a baby—especially if it's your sister's or sister's-in-law—can be really hard, as can the showers, christenings or baptisms, and the first birthday parties that go with it. The birth of a second or third child of friends who started trying about the same time as you can also be difficult. For women, there can be an added dimension with the arrival of menopause.

You can't avoid these things, but you can manage them. You can be aware that an anniversary is coming up, and acknowledge that you might not feel so good on that day. You can plan to take a day's leave, have a special dinner together, do something fun, or gentle, or nurturing. You can decline an invitation to a shower and choose not to visit a new mother and her baby in hospital. You can still send flowers, write a card, buy a present or make a phone call, any of which enable you to express your congratulations without making it harder on yourself. You can choose to go away for Christmas—just the two of you—and not attend the usual full-on family function with parents, babies and kids. It's about you now, and your needs as a couple—do what's best for you.

Rituals and memorials

As with any significant loss it can help to identify a particular day as a day of remembrance or memorial—a day when you allow yourselves to think about what you've been through, a day when you grieve for everything that was lost, everything that never was. This is a way of honouring your own experience and moving through the natural processes of grief. Maybe it's one day a month at first, then one day every six months and, eventually, once a year. It's an opportunity for you to think, to cry, to get angry or just to quietly

> The thought of not being a Dad didn't come upon me until somewhere around the third miscarriage. We were having rows and it was hard. I got to thinking, 'What do I think about that?' At the time I was numb. I was just really distraught about Lee. Then a friend said to me that he'd decided not to have children, but that he imagined when he was older he'd regret not having them. It matched how I felt perfectly. It was more than regret. I really do want children. I really did want children. It's a great empty hole, and I feel, like Lee, quite resigned that it's not going to happen. I just know how much I enjoy my own family, my own parents, and how I've got to know them as an adult and how important that is in my life, and to think that I won't be able to have that. It's a huge blow. Devastating really.
>
> Mark

> It was then that what I was facing crushed me [stopping trying to conceive]. I would have kept trying, but seeing Lee after a miscarriage . . . seeing the loss, the devastation. By the fourth time it was clear I couldn't ask her to go through that again.
>
> Mark

> I imagine building a place in the bush, healing myself and being open to the world and maybe wonderful things are still out there as I once believed. There will be. It will just take a bit more time.
>
> Mark

reflect. It can be a good way of helping you to focus your emotions and express them within a particular, specified timeframe, to prevent them from spilling into all the other days of the year.

Some people develop rituals which can be enormously comforting while you are working through your grief. One woman allocated a part of her garden where, once a month, after her period, she planted something as a memorial to her loss. Another created a patchwork quilt, adding a square each month. One couple bought flowers and floated them down a local river, another had a special dinner together. The expression of grief is an important part of the healing process—getting it out means it doesn't build up inside.

In other circumstances when you experience a loss, you might receive flowers, a card from a friend, or a call from a family member. People acknowledge your pain and try to help you through it. With infertility this doesn't always happen; your grief is less visible, more difficult to understand, and the support may not be forthcoming. Even if people want to be supportive, they may not know how to respond in a way that is going to make you feel better. You might find that as a couple you rely on each other more during this time, you feel that only your partner really understands what you are going through. Even then, there will be some things you can't share, and you will carry these alone. This is a time to be especially good to yourself and each other. Buy yourselves a bunch of flowers, send each other a card, phone unexpectedly.

> I just became more and more certain that I needed to do something different and that this [volunteering overseas] was really one of my dreams. To keep a sense of self, and self worth, I needed to follow one of my dreams, and I needed to find a way of letting go of another dream [being a mother] that I wasn't going to have and that was an important part of the healing process.
>
> Lee

Meeting your needs in other ways

Most people, when they decide to have children, don't really analyse *why* they want to have children. They might just have a sense that the timing is right, they feel ready. When you are facing a life without children, ironically, it can be helpful to try to understand

It's sad not to have kids, but it is also important to be okay in myself, to get to like my body again and to feel okay as Lee and not to struggle and get stuck in something that just wasn't possible. And it was really important to step outside myself because my world had got pretty narrow. It was really important to put my experience, my pain and Mark's pain, in a bigger picture and say, 'You don't always get what you want and that's okay'. It's tragic for Mark and I, but in the bigger scheme of things it's a small drop in the ocean.

Lee

We talked about if it didn't happen and resigned ourselves to being childless, but we'd still be together forever and perhaps have a slightly different life. We'd be in the Andes or somewhere right now climbing up some mountain.

Greg

the reasons you wanted to have them in the first place. Those needs don't go away just because you stop trying. If you can identify the needs that would have been fulfilled by having a child, you can start to develop other ways of meeting them.

Commonly, these needs include the need to pass on genetic material—to see ourselves reflected in our children—the need to pass on the family name and fulfil a role in our own families, the need to create or nurture or to pass on certain values, the need to give and receive love. These needs can sometimes be met through relationships with other children, particularly nephews and nieces, or the kids of close friends; the role of uncle or aunt can be extremely rewarding. Sometimes these needs can be met through contact with kids in different social environments—coaching a sports team, being a big brother/sister in a buddy scheme, volunteering to help with the local school camp. Sometimes—though perhaps not as often as people expect—they can be met through adoption or fostering (see below).

> I've done five years of study over the period of treatment, so I guess that was my outlet—something completely different and unrelated to my work. I've been studying horticulture and I now work one day a week in that industry. I absolutely love it. It was never a field I thought would have interested me—I always imagined that I would be in an office—and yet here I am planting out these pretty little petunias, and pansies and things like that. I'm interested to see how they will grow, a kind of nurturing, so there is a relationship with all this stuff, I suppose.
>
> Tanya

> I was thinking over the weekend when I was aunty-ing my nephews. I want to be part of kids' lives. I really enjoy them and that's really bitter-sweet. Different people find their own way of healing. The grief that I feel, I don't think it will ever go away because there are constant reminders, you know: babysitting my nephews, or seeing other people with kids, or seeing other people pregnant and knowing that it's something that won't be part of my life experience. It's very sad. It is also about trying to find other things that are important, to contribute, to try to be as engaged as I can and participate in the world in as honest a way as possible. And that may mean just being a friend, or a lover, or an aunty, or a worker, or a member of a community, and it may not mean being a mother and that's okay.
>
> Lee

Different types of nurturing

Many infertile couples, however, do not meet these needs solely through relationships with children, but find other ways to meet them. Some people include nurturing and growth in their lives by focusing on the land, the environment, or animals. One couple, for example, bought a block of land in the country and planted and nurtured a native forest. They bought a few farm animals and set up a camp for kids from the city. One couple went to South America where the woman photographed butterflies, and the man wrote a book about them. Another couple became involved in the redevelopment of local parkland which included organising clean-up and tree-planting days for kids. Some people explore their creativity in broadly artistic ways: writing a book, taking an art class, learning carpentry, joining a choir, making sculpture, writing poetry, learning a musical instrument, dressmaking or quilting, building a shed or an extension, taking up photography.

No one is suggesting that any of these things make up for not having a child, but they can help to meet some of your needs in the difficult time that follows a decision to stop trying for a family. They can give you a sense of putting something in and getting something back. They can provide you with something that feels meaningful and worthwhile. Lots of people throw themselves into their work after they stop trying, which can be a distraction and a focus for energy. Some people take time out and go travelling. Both of these can help you move through the transition period between trying for a family and living without children, but they may not be sufficiently sustaining in the long term. Most people need something more than this. In the end, many people do, in fact, find rewarding ways of spending the additional time they have as a result of not having children.

Adoption

At some stage during the time you are trying to conceive, you will invariably be asked whether you have thought of adopting. This is often presented as both an obvious solution to your problem and an

Ages ago we got all the forms and had a read through the adoption stuff. I guess that's part of the reason why, especially in the last year, we really wanted to set a time limit to our treatment. Charles has always been much closer to adopting than me . . . I sort of had to work my way there. I said, 'January next year, we'll seriously consider it as an option.' But then donor eggs came up which we sort of hadn't considered as so much of an option, and we thought maybe that's a good option. But we have pretty much stuck to our timeline which has made it easier.

Hannah

I guess we are lucky because we are only 30 now, even though we don't feel young, everyone keeps telling us we are young for IVF and for adoption. That's why I think you really have to decide what is important: is it raising a child or having a child who is biologically connected to you? I guess you have to decide what you want.

Charles

easy option, when in most cases it is neither. Adopting is not necessarily the next logical step after unsuccessful attempts to have children, as is often suggested. There are a number of reasons for this. In Australia at the moment, very few babies come up for adoption, and it can take many years for a baby to become available—the numbers are just so small. You may be able to adopt an older child, or a child who has special needs because of a disability, but this is a very different experience from adopting an infant with whom you can bond immediately and form a lasting attachment. These days, also, local adoptions often involve the child having ongoing contact with the birth mother.

For many couples, age may also be a factor, especially if they have spent a number of years trying to conceive unsuccessfully, or have experienced recurrent miscarriage. The process of being assessed and accepted as potential adopting parents can take a number of years. If you have already gone through years of treatment or trying you might not want to put yourself through another complex and protracted process. Adopting from overseas may be an option, but again it is not that simple (see below). It also takes a very long time, and the significant costs involved put it out of reach of many people.

Having said all that, adoption *is* possible and can be a very positive solution for some people. Providing a loving home for a child who might otherwise not have one can be enormously rewarding and you can, finally, create your own family. Many couples have successfully moved through IVF to adoption.

Local adoption

Australian adoptions are managed by the community or welfare services department in your state or territory (contact details are listed in 'Information and resources'). In addition, there are a number of private agencies that handle adoptions. The criteria for selection vary from state to state and from agency to agency. If you are thinking about adopting, it is worth making some initial enquiries early to make sure you don't miss out. Some departments or agencies have age restrictions, some may require you are married, or in a de facto relationship, or have been together for a certain length of time. Some consider applications from single people. Applications from lesbian and gay couples are not accepted, though you might, possibly, be able to apply as a single person and would be a fair way down the pecking order.

Most departments have regulations relating to requests from people who are having, or have had, fertility treatment. Some agencies will not let you apply while you are still having treatment and require a six-month gap between stopping treatment and lodging your application. The agencies will normally send out introductory information on request, or you can access it online. Most run information sessions where you can find out how it all works and ask questions.

Adopting from overseas

Most overseas adoptions are managed by the same government welfare departments and are often organised with specific countries they have established a relationship with. There are also some private agencies. If you give them a call they will send you some introductory information and details of information sessions you can attend. You may have a greater chance of adopting an infant if you adopt from overseas, but it is a long and complex process and, for many people, the costs are prohibitive. With overseas adoptions there are a whole range of additional issues around culture, language, race and ethnicity that you have to address. Though the numbers are still small, some Australian families have successfully and happily adopted children from overseas.

Fostering

Fostering may be an option for some people who have come to the end of their own attempts to create a family. It is a way of having contact with children, of providing care and affection, and of having a parental role. Foster care can be provided for a few days, a few weeks, a few months or longer. Fostering is handled through state or territory family or welfare departments and a number of private agencies. All potential foster parents have to go through a fairly lengthy and detailed assessment process. Eligibility requirements vary, though the criteria are not usually as strict as for adoption. Details can be accessed online or mailed out to you. Most agencies consider applications from de-facto couples and from single people. Some agencies welcome applications from lesbians and gay men.

Summing up

- Stopping treatment can be a difficult time, but it can also offer some relief as you begin to regain control over your life. Your focus can shift to new and different things and you can start to plan again.
- There will be all sorts of things—particularly days and special events—that will remind you of your infertility and will make you think of 'what might have been'. Although you cannot change what has happened, you can do things to help manage the difficult time after stopping treatment.
- Many people develop rituals or personal ways of acknowledging what they have been through which can help in the process of grieving.
- Becoming involved with children in other ways, developing an interest in the land, the environment or animals, or exploring artistic or creative interests can help to deal with the sense of loss.
- Some people are able to adopt successfully—either within Australia, or overseas—and some find fostering rewarding.

Final thoughts

Throughout the time you are dealing with infertility and its treatment, you will undoubtedly receive lots of advice and suggestions from well-meaning friends and family. The most important thing of all, however, is to do what's right for you. If that means boycotting Christmas or declining to attend yet another baby shower, if it means getting your chakras realigned or seeing a hypnotherapist, if it means staying in bed all day eating Tim Tams or watching reruns of Oprah—if it means stripping the car down again or repainting the lounge room, or ignoring your friends for a while and going to the gym every night—then so be it. If there was ever a time to be a little selfish, this is it. However you handle your particular situation, never forget that this is a huge, complex and difficult thing no one ever prepared you for. Be kind to each other. Be gentle on yourselves.

Information and resources

Infertility clinics

Australian Capital Territory

Canberra Fertility Centre
John James Memorial Hospital
Strickland Crescent
Deakin ACT 2600
Tel: (02) 6282 5458
Fax: (02) 6281 2087
Website: *www.canberrafertility-center.com.au*

Sydney IVF Canberra
Suite 16, John James Medical Centre
175 Strickland Cresent
Deakin ACT 2600
Tel: (02) 6260 3400
Fax: (02) 6260 3466
Email: *canberra@sivf.com.au*

New South Wales

IVF Australia
IVF Australia includes North Shore ART, City West IVF, IVF South and IVF East
Website: *www.ivf.com.au*

North Shore ART
Level 1, 24 Thomas Street
Chatswood NSW 2067
Tel: (02) 9904 8900
Fax: (02) 9904 8911
Email:
mail@northshorefertility.com.au
Website: *www.nsart.com.au*

City West IVF
City West House
12 Caroline Street
Westmead NSW 2145
Tel: (02) 9689 1966
Fax: (02) 9633 3730
Email: *citywest@ivf.com.au*
Website: *www.ivf.com.au*

IVF South
St George Private Medical Complex
South Street
Kogarah NSW 2217
Tel: (02) 9553 7555
Fax: (02) 9553 7886
Email: *ivfs@ivfsouth.com.au*
Website: *www.ivfsouth.com.au*

IVF East
PO Box 51
Randwick NSW 2031
Tel: (02) 9382 6686
Fax: (02) 9382 6587
Email: *ivf@doctor.com*
Website: *www.ivf-east.com*

Sydney IVF
Level 2, 4 O'Connell Street
Sydney NSW 2000
Tel: (02) 9221 5964
Fax: (02) 9233 7519
Email: *reception@sivf.com.au*
Website: *www.sivf.com.au*

Westmead Fertility Centre
Westmead Hospital
Tel: (02) 9845 7484
Fax: (02) 9845 7793
Website: *www.westmeadivf.com.au*

IVF New South Wales
Level 3, 253 Oxford Street
Bondi Junction NSW 2022
Tel: (02) 9389 0927
Fax: (02) 9387 8580

King George V Hospital
Level 6 North, Fertility Ward
Missendon Road
Camperdown NSW 2050
Tel: (02) 9515 8824
Fax: (02) 9515 7976

Sydney IVF Newcastle
23 Merewether Street
Merewether NSW 2291
Tel: (02) 4969 6342
Fax: (02) 4965 3721
Email: *reception@sivf.com.au*
Website: *www.sivf.com.au*

Albury Reproductive Medicine Centre
1084 Pemberton Stret
Albury NSW 2640
Tel: (02) 6041 2677
Fax: (02) 6041 2118
Website: *www.reproductivemedicine.com.au*

Fertility First
Centre for Reproductive Health
Hurstville Community Hospital
Level 1, 2 Pearl Street
Hurstville NSW 2220
Tel: (02) 9586 3311
Fax: (02) 9586 3322

Email: *fert1@fertilityfirst.com.au*
Website: *www.fertilityfirst.com.au*

Northern Territory

Repromed
Reproductive Medicine Unit
Darwin Private Hospital
Rocklands Drive
Tiwi NT 0810
Tel: (08) 8945 4211
Fax: (08) 8945 4255
Email: *darwin@repromed.com.au*
Website: *www.repromed.com.au*

Queensland

Monash IVF
25 Spendelove Avenue
Southport QLD 4215
Tel: (07) 5532 0169
Fax: (07) 5591 9403
Email: *info@monashivf.edu.au*
Website: *www.monashivf.edu.au*

Queensland Fertility Group
Watkins Medical Centre
1st Floor, 225 Wickham Terrace
Brisbane QLD 4000
Tel: (07) 3832 4262
Fax: (07) 3832 7790
Website: *www.qfg.com.au*

The Wesley IVF Service
Wesley Medical Centre
Chaseley Street
Auchenflower QLD 4066
Tel: (07) 3232 7088
Fax: (07) 3870 7810
Email: *wivf.clinic@wesley.com.au*
Website: *www.ivf.wesley.com.au*

North Queensland IVF Services
Suite 5, 1st Floor
Park Haven Medical Centre
7 Bayswater Road
Townsville QLD 4812
Tel: (07) 4722 1299
Fax: (07) 4721 4600

Queensland Fertility Group—Toowoomba
Suite 15, 9 Scott Street
Toowoomba QLD 4350
Tel: (07) 4638 5243
Fax: (07) 4639 1652

Monash IVF Queensland
Suite 12, 259 McCullough Street
Sunnybank QLD 4109
Tel: (07) 3345 4455
Fax: (07) 3345 4466
Email: *info@monashivf.edu.au*
Website: *www.monashivf.edu.au*

South Australia

Reproductive Medicine Unit
Queen Elizabeth Hospital
28 Woodville Rd
Woodville SA 5011
Tel: (08) 8222 6782
Fax: (08) 8222 6080
Email: *qeh@repromed.com.au*
Website: *www.repromed.com.au*

Reproductive Medicine Unit
Wakefield Clinic
Level 1, 270 Wakefield Street

Adelaide SA 5000
Tel: (08) 8232 5100
Fax: (08) 8224 0337
Email: *wakefield@repromed.com.au*
Website: *www.repromed.com.au*

Reproductive Medicine Programme
Flinders Medical Centre
Bedford Park SA 5042
Tel: (08) 8204 4343
Fax: (08) 8204 5454
Email: *enquire@flindersivf.com.au*
Website: *www.flindersivf.com.au*

Tasmania

Sydney IVF—Launceston
No. 10, 11 High Street
Launceston TAS 7250
Tel: (03) 6335 3380
Fax: (03) 6335 3381

Tas IVF
St Helen's Private Hospital
186 Macquarie Street
Hobart TAS 7000
Tel: (03) 6221 6501
Fax: (03) 6223 4996
Email: *tasivf@trump.net.au*

Victoria

Melbourne IVF
Suite 10, 320 Victoria Parade
East Melbourne VIC 3002
Tel: (03) 9473 4444
Fax: (03) 9473 4454
Website: *www.mivf.com.au*

Reproductive Biology Unit
Royal Women's Hospital
132 Grattan Street
Carlton VIC 3053
Tel: (03) 9344 2372
Fax: (03) 9349 1387

Monash IVF—Clayton
252 Clayton Road
Clayton VIC 3168
Tel: (03) 9543 2833
Fax: (03) 9548 9150
Email: *info@monashivf.edu.au*
Website: *www.monashivf.edu.au*

Monash IVF—Richmond
4th Floor, Epworth Hospital
89 Bridge Rd
Richmond VIC 3121
Tel: (03) 9429 9188
Fax: (03) 9427 1973
Email: *info@monashivf.edu.au*
Website: *www.monashivf.edu.au*

Melbourne Assisted Conception Centre
2nd Level, St Francis Building
166 Gipps Street
East Melbourne VIC 3002
Tel: (03) 9270 2674
Fax: (03) 9270 2673
Email: *macc_talbot@hotmail.com*
Website:
www.assistedconception.com.au

Mildura Reproductive Medicine
4 Healthscope Court
Mildura VIC 3500
Tel: (03) 5021 4898
Fax: (03) 5021 4405

Western Australia

Concept Fertility Centre
374 Bagot Rd
Subiaco WA 6008
Tel: (08) 9382 2388
Fax: (08) 9381 3603
Email: *concept@conceptfert.com.au*
Website: *www.conceptfert.com.au*

Pivet Medical Centre
166–168 Cambridge Street
West Leederville WA 6007
Tel: (08) 9382 1677
Fax: (08) 9382 4576
Email: *pivetmc@iinet.net.au*
Website: *www.pivet.com.au*

Support groups

Most IVF clinics have local support groups run by current or former patients. Support groups provide an opportunity to meet and talk with other people who have infertility problems and who are undergoing treatment. Most groups organise social functions, run information sessions, and produce and distribute a local newsletter to members. Some groups have their own website—or a page on the official clinic website—or you can access their contact details directly from the clinic. There are also some national and statewide organisations that provide a broad range of services and support and promote the interests of people with infertility problems through representation and advocacy at a national level.

The Australian and New Zealand Infertility Cousellors Association
Website:
www.swin.edu.au/hosting/anzica/ANZIChome.htm

Access—Australia's National Infertility Network
PO Box 959
Parramatta NSW 2124
Tel: (02) 9670 2380
Fax: (02) 9670 2638
Email: *info@access.org.au*
Website: *www.access.org.au*

Oasis Infertility Support Inc.
GPO Box 2420
Adelaide SA 5001
Tel: (08) 8223 7434
Email: *oasissupport@chariot.net.au*
Website:
www.users.chariot.net.au/~oasissupport

Genesis Infertility Support Group
Box 1574
Booragoon WA 6154

Tel: (08) 9375 7572
Website:
www.users.bigpond.com/genesissup-port

Friends of Queensland Fertility Group
GPO Box 1271
Brisbane QLD 4001
Email: *friendsqfg@rocketmail.com*
Website:
www.geocities.com/hotsprings/2952

Donor Conception Support Group of Australia
PO Box 53
Georges Hall NSW 2198
Email: *dcsg@optushome.com.au*
Website:
http://members.optushome.com.au/dcsg

Australian Multiple Birth Association
PO Box 105
Coogee NSW 2034
Email:
amba_national@yahoo.com.au
Website: *www.amba.org.au*

Endometriosis Association
28 Warrandyte Road
Ringwood VIC 3134
Tel: (03) 9879 2199
Fax: (03) 9879 6519
Email: *info@endometriosis.org.au*
Website: *www.endometriosis.org.au*

Polycystic Ovarian Syndrome Association of Australia
PO Box 689
Kingswood NSW 2747
Tel: (02) 8250 0222
Email: *info@posaa.asn.au*
Website: *www.posaa.asn.au*

Quit—The National Tobacco Campaign
Tel: (02) 6289 1555
Email: *quitnow@health.gov.au*
Website: *www.quitnow.info.au*

Prospective lesbian parenting support groups

Most states have some kind of prospective lesbian parenting support group. They are generally fairly informal, run by a few women who organise meetings and maybe send out an occasional newsletter. Contact numbers are usually their private home or mobile phone, and they can change frequently. You might have to ask around to find out what is available in your area. You could start with your local lesbian and gay switchboard, check the local gay press, or ask at a women's health or community centre.

Fostering and adoption

Australian Capital Territory

Family Services
PO Box 1584
Tuggeranong ACT 2901
Tel: (02) 6207 1080
Fax: (02) 6207 8888
Email: *decs.webmaster@act.gov.au*
Website: *www.decs.act.gov.au*

New South Wales

Department of Community Services
Adoption Services
PO Box 3485
Parramatta NSW 2124
Tel: (02) 9865 5904
Fax: (02) 9689 3587
Email:
adoption@community.nsw.gov.au
Website:
www.community.nsw.gov.au

Northern Territory

Department of Health and Community Services
Adoptions Unit
PO Box 40596
Casuarina
Darwin NT 0811
Tel: (08) 8922 7077
Fax: (08) 8922 7480
Website: *www.nt.gov.au*

Queensland

Department of Families, Youth and Community Care
Adoption Services
GPO Box 806
Brisbane QLD 4001
Tel: (07) 3224 8045
Fax: (07) 3404 3570
Email: *mailbox@families.qld.gov.au*
Website: *www.families.qld.gov.au*

South Australia

Department of Human Services
Adoption and Family Information Service
PO Box 287
Rundle Mall
Adelaide SA 5000
Tel: (08) 8207 0060
Fax: (08) 8226 6974
Email: *adoptions@saugov.sa.gov.au*
Website: *www.dhs.sa.gov.au*

Tasmania

Department of Health and Human Services
Adoption and Information Service
PO Box 538
Hobart TAS 7001
Tel: (03) 6222 7373
Fax: (03) 6223 1343
Email:
adoption.services@dhhs.tas.gov.au
Website:*www.dchs.tas.gov.au*

Victoria

Department of Human Services and Community Care
PO Box 4057
Melbourne VIC 3001
Phone: (03) 9616 7232
Fax: (03) 9616 7974
Email:
community.care@dhs.vic.gov.au
Website: *www.dhs.vic.gov.au*

Western Australia

Department for Community Development
Adoption Services
PO Box 6334
East Perth WA 6004
Tel: (08) 9222 2555
Tel: 1800 622 258
TTY: (08) 9325 1232
Fax (08) 9222 2607
Website: *www.dcd.wa.gov.au*

Australian Inter Country Adoption Network
PO Box 7420
Bondi Beach NSW 2026
Tel: (02) 9371 9244
Fax: (02) 9371 9544
Email: *affc@ihug.com.au*

Medical associations

The Royal Australian and New Zealand College of Obstetricians and Gynaecologists (RANZCOG)
College House
254 Albert Street
East Melbourne VIC 3002
Tel: (03) 9417 1699
Fax: (03) 9419 0672
Email: *ranzcog@ranzcog.edu.au*
Website: *www.ranzcog.edu.au*

National Health and Medical Research Council (NHMRC)
GPO Box 9848
Canberra ACT 2601
Tel: (02) 6289 9184
Fax: (02) 6289 9197
Email: *exec.sec@nhmrc.gov.au*
Website: *www.nhmrc.gov.au*

Fertility Society of Australia
Waldron Smith Management
61 Danks Street
Port Melbourne VIC 3207
Tel:(03) 9645 6359
Fax:(03) 9645 6322
Email: *wscn@convention.net.au*
Website: *www.fsa.au.com*

Legislation and legal bodies

Reproductive Technology Act, 1988 (South Australia)
South Australian Council on Reproductive Technology
Department of Human Services
PO Box 287 Rundle Mall
Adelaide SA 5000
Tel: (08) 8226 6048
Fax: (08) 8226 6778
Website: *www.dhs.sa.gov.au*

Infertility Treatment Act, 1995 (Victoria)
Infertility Treatment Authority
Level 30
570 Bourke Street
Melbourne VIC 3000
Tel: (03) 8601 5250
Fax: (03) 8601 5277
Email: *ita@ita.org.au*
Website: *www.ita.org.au*

Human Reproductive Technology Act, 1991 (Western Australia)
Reproductive Technology Council
189 Royal Street
East Perth WA 6004
Tel: (08) 9222 4260
Fax: (08) 9222 4236
Email: *sandy.webb@health.wa.gov.au*
Website: *http://numbat.murdoch.edu.au/RTC/rtchome.html*

Sex Discrimination Act, 1984 (Cth)
Human Rights and Equal Opportunity Commission (HREOC)
Level 8, Piccadilly Tower
133 Castlereagh Street
Sydney NSW 2000
Tel: (02) 9284 9600 or 1300 369 711
Fax: (02) 9284 9611
TTY: 1800 620 241
Email: *paffairs@humanrights.gov.au*
Website: *www.hreoc.gov.au*

General information websites

A note on using the Internet for general information

A search of 'IVF' or 'infertility' will generate hundreds of websites that provide information about various medical conditions, drugs, procedures and treatments. Other sites describe the experiences of people undergoing treatment and explore the emotional ups and downs. There are also IVF chat rooms where you can talk online with other people who have fertility problems. Most of the sites provide reliable and up-to-date information, but it is wise to approach some with a little caution. Be wary, for example, of those that offer medical advice or make claims of scientific breakthroughs or new treatments. Stick with the clinic websites, the various government and medical bodies, the individual associations for specific conditions and the support groups.

The International Council on Infertility Information Dissemination, Inc.
www.inciid.org

Infertility Consumer Support for Infertility (iCSi)
www.icsi.ws

Ferti.Net: Worldwide Fertility Network
www.ferti.net

Electronic Infertility Network
www.ein.org

FertAid
www.fertaid.com

International Federation of Fertility Societies (IFFS)
www.mnet.fr/iffs

American Society for Reproductive Medicine
www.asrm.org

European Society for Human Reproduction & Embryology
www.eshre.com

British Fertility Society
www.britishfertilitysociety.org.uk

The American Infertility Association
www.americaninfertility.org

The Bertarelli Foundation
www.bertarelli.edu

www.fertilityworld.org

Glossary

Adhesions: scar tissue, usually from earlier surgery or infection, that can obstruct the movement of egg or sperm

Agglutination: when sperm clump together, rather than moving freely

Agonist: a synthetic hormone that briefly stimulates the *pituitary gland* to release *follicle stimulating hormone* (FSH) and *lutenising hormone* (LH), but then suppresses their production

Amenorrhoea: where a woman has no menstrual periods

Androgens: male sex hormones—testosterone is the main androgen in men and androgens are also present in small amounts in women

Andrologist: a specialist in male reproductive health

Aneuploidy: an incorrect number of chromosomes that results in abnormalities

Anovulation: where a woman does not ovulate

Antagonist: a synthetic hormone that immediately stops the *pituitary gland* releasing *follicle stimulating hormone* (FSH) and *lutenising hormone* (LH)

Antiphospholipid antibodies: antibodies that may be associated with tiny blood clots forming in the blood vessels of the placenta, and which may be associated with miscarriage

Anti-sperm antibodies: antibodies that can attach to the head or tail of the sperm and, in sufficient numbers, make it difficult for the sperm to fertilise the egg

Artificial insemination (AI): when sperm is inserted into the vagina or uterus, normally with a syringe or catheter; AI may be either artificial insemination by husband (AIH) or artificial insemination by donor (AID) (also known as donor insemination (DI)

Artificial thaw cycle: a treatment protocol using thawed embryos and some low-level drug treatment to prepare the uterus to accept a pregnancy

Asherman's syndrome: a condition where the sides of the uterus start to grow together, usually as a result of scarring from previous infection or surgery, and cause damage to the endometrium

Aspermia: where a man has no semen

Assisted hatching: a process of artificially puncturing the outer shell of an embryo to help it 'hatch'

Asthenozoospermia: where the sperm is weak and has poor motility

Azoospermia: where a man has no sperm

Basal body temperature: the temperature of the body which can be tracked to assist in identifying whether ovulation has occurred

Bicornuate uterus: a congenital condition in which both the inside and outside of the uterus are divided

Biochemical pregnancy: when a blood test shows evidence of raised *human chorionic gonadotropin* (HCG) levels, but there is no ongoing clinical pregnancy

Blastocyst: the stage of the embryo, about five days after it has fertilised, when it usually implants into the lining of the uterus

Blighted ovum: where there is a gestational sac, but no evidence of a foetus

Catheter: a fine plastic tube used for transferring embryos and for other procedures

Cervical mucus: mucus secreted by the cervix around the time of ovulation to help the movement of sperm

Cervix: the neck of the uterus

Cetrotide: a brand name of a gonadotropin-releasing hormone-antagonist

Chlamydia: a micro-organism that can be sexually transmitted and may cause infection and adhesions in the pelvis

Chromosomes: thread-like structures that appear in pairs in human cells and carry genetic material

Cilia: fine hair-like structures in the fallopian tube that help move the egg

Cleavage: the process by which a fertilised egg divides

Clomid: brand name of the drug clomiphene

Clomiphene: a drug that increases the natural production of *follicle stimulating hormone* (FSH)

Clomiphene cycle: a treatment protocol involving low-level follicle stimulation using the drug clomiphene

Comparative genome hybridisation (CGH): a new technique for assessing the embryos before they are transferred, a form of pre-implantation genetic diagnosis

Complete abortion: where all the products of contraception have passed out of the body naturally after a miscarriage

Corpus luteum: the structure that remains after the egg has left the follicle, which is responsible for producing progesterone to support a pregnancy in its early stages

Cryptorchidism: a condition where the testes do not descend into the scrotum

Curette: a procedure to remove tissue from the uterus, usually referred to with 'dilation'—a 'D and C'

Cyst: a sac or structure containing fluid or other matter

Cystic fibrosis: a serious genetic disorder that affects the development of the lungs

Cytomegalovirus (CMV): a virus that can be transmitted via semen

Cytoplasm: the part of an egg that surrounds the nucleus into which the sperm is injected in the process of *intracytoplasmic sperm injection* (ICSI)

Depo provera: a long acting injectible contraceptive

Dilation: an 'opening', usually referring to the opening of the cervix in order to perform a curette—a 'D and C'

Down regulated protocol: a treatment protocol involving the gradual suppression of natural hormones with a *GnRH-agonist* and the stimulation of follicles with a *follicle stimulating hormone* (FSH)

Downs syndrome: a genetic disease caused by an extra chromosome 21, also known as *trisomy 21*

Dysmenorrhea: a condition in which a woman has painful periods

Ectopic pregnancy: where a pregnancy forms outside the uterus, normally in the fallopian tube

Egg pick-up: the commonly used term for *ovum pick-up*

Ejaculate: the seminal fluid that is expelled from the penis during ejaculation

Ejaculatory duct: part of the male reproductive system attached to the seminal vesicle

Embryo: a fertilised egg

Embryo transfer (ET): the process of transferring an embryo that has been created *in vitro* into the uterus

Endocrinology: the study of hormones

Endometriosis: a condition in which endometrial tissue grows in places other than in the uterus

Endometritis: a condition where the endometrium becomes inflamed

Endometrium: the lining of the uterus which sheds as menstruation (period)

Epididymis: a part of the male reproductive system in which sperm are stored and nourished

Epididymitis: a condition where the epididymis becomes inflamed

Fallopian tube: part of the female reproductive system, connecting the ovaries to the uterus

Fibroid: a non-cancerous tumour that can form in the uterus

Fimbria: tiny finger-like structures at the open end of the fallopian tube that 'pick-up' the egg once it has been released from the ovary

Flare protocol: a treatment protocol that involves less suppression of natural hormones and takes advantage of the body's flare of *follicle stimulating hormone* (FSH) and *lutenising hormone* (LH) caused by the agonist before it becomes suppressive

Foetal alcohol syndrome: a condition that newborn babies are born with as a result of excessive alcohol intake by the mother during pregnancy

Follicle: a sac in the ovary that contains an egg

Follicle stimulating hormone (FSH): a hormone produced by the pituitary gland—in women it stimulates follicles on the ovaries to grow and in men it stimulates the production of sperm in the testes

Follicular phase: the first part of the menstrual cycle, before ovulation

Fragile X syndrome: a syndrome of impaired functioning in males, which often causes mental retardation

Fundus: the main part of the uterus, particularly the top area away from the cervix

Gamete: sperm or egg

Gamete intrafallopian transfer (GIFT): a procedure where eggs are retrieved, mixed with sperm and then inserted into the fallopian tube

Gonadotropin releasing hormone (GnRH): a hormone produced by the hypothalamus that regulates the production of *follicle stimulating hormone* (FSH) and lutenising hormone (LH)

Gonadotrophin releasing hormone-agonist: see *agonist*

Gonadotrophin releasing hormone-antagonist: see *antagonist*

Gonal F: a brand name of a synthetic follicle stimulating hormone

Gonorrhoea: a bacterial infection that can be sexually transmitted

Haemophilia: a sex-linked genetic disease of the blood

Hepatitis B and C: infectious diseases that cause inflammation of the liver

Herpes: a sexually transmitted viral disease

Hormone: a natural chemical substance passed into the blood that stimulates organs to action

Huntington's disease: a genetic disorder that is associated with deterioration in functioning, often in one's thirties and forties

Human chorionic gonadotropin (HCG): a hormone secreted by the placenta during pregnancy, the presence of which shows up on a pregnancy test; also sometimes given as luteal support under the brand name Pregnyl or Profasi

Human immune-deficiency virus (HIV): a sexually transmitted virus that causes acquired immune deficiency syndrome (AIDS)

Hydrosalpinx: when fluid develops on the fallopian tube because of a blockage

Hyperprolactinaemia: where too much prolactin is produced by the pituitary gland

Hypothalmic anovulation: where there is no ovulation because the hypothalmus doesn't produce sufficient *gonadotropin releasing hormone* (GnRH) or the pituitary doesn't respond to stimulation with *GnRH*

Hypothalmus: a part of the brain that controls the *pituitary gland*, and which is responsible for producing gonadotropin releasing hormone (GnRH)

Hysterosalpingogram (HSG): an x-ray procedure for examining the endometrial cavity and internal outline of the fallopian tubes

Hysteroscopy: an exploratory procedure for examining the uterine cavity using a fine telescope-like instrument, similar to that used for a *laparoscopy*

Idiopathic infertility: where the cause of infertility is unknown

Immunobead test: a test carried out on sperm to check for the presence of anti-sperm antibodies

Implantation: where an embryo embeds itself into the lining of the uterus

Impotence: where a man is unable to maintain an erection

Incomplete abortion: where the products of conception do not pass out of the body naturally after a miscarriage

Intracytoplasmic sperm injection (ICSI): a technique for injecting a single sperm into an egg

Intramural fibroid: a fibroid that grows within the uterus wall

Intrauterine contraceptive device (IUD): a device inserted into the uterus as a method of contraception

Intrauterine insemination (IUI): a procedure in which sperm is inserted into the uterus using a catheter

In vitro fertilisation: the process of fertilising an egg in a laboratory

Isthmus: the part of the fallopian tube closest to the uterus

Karyotype: a systematised diagram of chromosomes

Klinefelters syndrome: a genetic condition in which a man has an extra X chromosome

Kremer test: a test that examines the interaction between sperm and cervical mucus

Laparoscopy: an exploratory surgical procedure for examining a woman's internal reproductive organs, performed under general anaesthetic

Laparotomy: a surgical operation on the abdomen

Leuprolide: the brand name of a GnRH agonist

LH surge: the increase in lutenising hormone that occurs in women just before ovulation

Listeria: a bacteria found in some foods that is very occasionally associated with pregnancy loss

Long protocol: another name for a 'down regulated' protocol

Lucrin (leuprolide): a brand name of a GnRH agonist

Luteal phase: the second half of the menstrual cycle, after ovulation

Luteal support: drugs given to help maintain the endometrium after an embryo transfer

Luteinising hormone (LH): a hormone secreted by the *pituitary gland*—responsible in women for ovulation of the mature follicle from the ovary

Menstrual cycle: a woman's reproductive cycle that involves the growth of follicles, release of eggs from the ovary, and the preparation of the lining of the uterus (the endometrium) to receive the eggs—normally about 26–34 days in length

Microgynon: the brand name of an oral contraceptive pill usually prescribed at the beginning of a stimulated treatment cycle to assist programming

Microsurgical epididymal sperm aspiration: a microsurgical procedure for retrieving sperm

Mid-luteal serum pregesterone: a blood test performed around day 21 of a woman's menstrual cycle to assess levels of progesterone

Miscarriage: when the foetus is lost before it is viable

Missed abortion: when there is a gestational sac and evidence of the foetus, but no heartbeat

Monosomy: where there is only one chromosome

Motility: the ability of sperm to move

Müllerian duct disorders: congenital defects of the female internal reproductive ducts which can result in abnormalities to the uterus and vagina

Myoma: a benign (non-cancerous) tumour of the muscle wall of the uterus, the same as a fibroid

Myomectomy: a surgical procedure performed to remove a fibroid/myoma

Myometrium: the muscle wall of the uterus

Natural thaw cycle: a treatment protocol that involves tracking natural ovulation and transferring a thawed embryo(s)

Oestradiol: the main naturally produced oestrogen

Oestrogen: female sex hormone responsible for stimulating growth

Oligomenorrhea: where a woman has menstrual cycles longer than 35 days

Oligoovulation: where a woman has infrequent ovulation

Oligozoospermia (oligospermia): where there is a reduced number of sperm in the ejaculate, 'a low sperm count'

Oocyte: an egg

Orchitis: an inflammation of the testes

Orgalutran: a brand name of a GnRH-antagonist

Ovarian cysts: a sac filled with fluid found in the ovary

Ovarian hyperstimulation syndrome: a condition where the ovaries become enlarged and fluid is released into the abdominal cavity

Ovary: female reproductive organ responsible for producing eggs

Ovulation: the release of egg(s) from the ovaries

Ovulation induction: where drugs are used to induce ovulation

Ovum (ova): an egg (eggs)

Ovum pick-up: where eggs are surgically retrieved from the ovaries, usually by transvaginal follicle aspiration

Pap smear: a test done to determine the presence of cancer cells or other abnormal cells in the cervix

Pelvic inflammatory disease (PID): an infection in the reproductive organs in a woman

Pessaries: a small tablet of a drug, in this case *progesterone*, that is inserted into the vagina

Pituitary gland: a gland controlled by the hypothalmus which is responsible for the production of *follicle stimulating hormone* (FSH) and *lutenising hormone* (LH) and other hormones

Polycystic ovarian syndrome (PCOS): a condition in women where there is a higher than normal production of the male hormone androgen, causing a range of symptoms that may affect fertility and often causes ovulatory difficulties

Polycystic ovaries (PCO): where a number of small cysts form on the ovaries, which may or may not affect fertility

Polyp: a benign (non-cancerous) growth of tissue

Post-coital test (PCT): a test used to determine sperm–mucus problems, increasingly replaced by the *Kremer test*

Pre-implantation genetic diagnosis (PGD): a technique for identifying genetic abnormalities in embryos before they are transferred into the uterus

Pregnyl: a brand name of a synthetic human chorionic gonadotropin (HCG)

Premature ovarian failure (POF): where a woman stops ovulating before the age of 40, also known as premature menopause

Primolut: a brand name of a progestagen

Products of conception: the gestational sac and foetal tissue remaining after a miscarriage

Profasi: a brand name of a synthetic *human chorionic gonadotropin* (HCG)

Progestagen: a progesterone-like substance, sometime used to regulate menstrual bleeding

Progesterone: a key female hormone secreted by the *corpus luteum* and responsible for supporting a pregnancy in its early stage

Prognyova: a brand name of an oestrogen

Prolactin: a hormone that stimulates the production of milk, disturbances of which can impair ovulation

Proliferative phase: the first half of the menstrual cycle, before ovulation

Proluton: a brand name for a progesterone injection

Pronuclei: the cells that form after a fertilised egg has divided

Prostatitis: infection of the prostate gland

Protocol: the combination of drugs and procedures for an IVF treatment cycle

Puregon: a brand name of a synthetic follicle stimulating hormone

Recurrent miscarriage: generally defined as three or more miscarriages in a row with no successful pregnancy in between

Retrogade ejaculation: where part of the ejaculate moves backwards into the bladder

Rubella (German measles): a disease which can cause developmental abnormalities in an unborn baby if contracted by the mother during pregnancy

Salpingitis: inflammation of the fallopian tubes

Salpingogram: an x-ray procedure used to examine the fallopian tubes

Scrotum: pouches of skin containing the testicles

Secretory phase: the second phase of the menstrual cycle, after ovulation

Secondary infertility: when a woman cannot conceive after already having had a pregnancy

Semen: the fluid produced at ejaculation

Seminal vesicles: male sex organs that contribute to the development of semen

Septate uterus: where a barrier (a septum) divides the uterus into two

Short protocol: another name for a flare protocol

Sickle cell anaemia: a genetic disease of the blood

Sonohysterogram: an ultrasound procedure for examining the endometrial cavity and internal outline of the fallopian tubes

Speculum: an instrument inserted into the vagina, used for pap smears, embryo transfers and inseminations

Sperm (spermatazoa): the male reproductive cell

Sperm–mucus penetration test: a technique for examining the interaction between sperm and cervical mucus (also known as the *Kremer test*)

Subcutaneous: under the skin

Submucous fibroid: a fibroid that grows inwards in the uterine cavity

Subserous fibroid: a fibroid that grows on the outside of the uterus

Surrogacy: when a woman carries a baby for someone else

Synarel: a brand name of an GnRH-agonist

Syphilis: a bacteria that can be sexually transmitted

Tay Sachs disease: a serious genetic disorder affecting the brain

Testes (testicles): the two male sex glands

Testicular biopsy: a surgical procedure where a small amount of tissue is removed from the testes to diagnose a fertility problem or to retrieve sperm

Testosterone: the main male sex hormone secreted in the testes and necessary for the development of sperm, also found in women in smaller quantities

Tetraozoospermia: where sperm are malformed or misshapen

Thalassemia: a genetic condition that affects the blood

Thyroid stimulating hormone: a hormone produced by the pituitary gland that activates the thyroid gland

Translocation: where part of a chromosome is knocked off and attaches to another chromosome

Transvaginal follicle aspiration: a technique for retrieving eggs during an IVF treatment cycle

Transvaginal ultrasound scan: a technique for examining a woman's internal reproductive organs, often used to monitor the development of follicles and the endometrium

'Trigger' injection: an injection of human chorionic gonadotropin (HCG) that activates ovulation

Trisomy: when there is an extra chromosome

Tubal patency: the extent to which the fallopian tubes are open

Ultrasound follicle aspiration: the medical term for ovum (egg) pick-up

Urethra: a tube which transport urine out of the body and, in men, is part of the sperm transport system

Uterus: the womb, where a pregnancy develops and gestates

Uterus didelphus: where there are two separate cavities in the uterus

Vaginismus: a condition where the muscles in the vagina spasm and make intercourse painful or difficult

Varicocele: small varicose veins that develop on the testes

Vas deferens: part of the male reproductive system that connects the epididymis with the seminal vesicles

Vasectomy: a male sterilisation procedure

Vasography: an x-ray procedure performed to examine the penis and testes

Vasovasostomy (vasoepididymostomy): the reversal of a vasectomy

Zona pellucida: the outer shell of an egg

Zygote: a fertilised egg before it divides for the first time

Further reading

Conception and pre-pregnancy

Dr Sarah Bremer, *Planning A Baby? How to prepare for a healthy pregnancy and give your baby the best possible start*, Vermillion, Ebury Press, Random House, UK, 1998.

Helen Caton, *The Fertility Plan: Your guide to conceiving a healthy baby*, Simon and Schuster, Australia, 2000.

Anne Charlish, *Getting Pregnant: How to improve your chances of a healthy conception*, Octopus Publishing Group, UK, 2002.

Kaz Cooke and Ruth Trickey, *Problem Periods: Natural and medical solutions*, Allen & Unwin, Australia, 2002.

D. S. Feingold and D. Gordon, *Getting Pregnant the Natural Way: The women's natural health series*, John Wiley and Sons inc., USA, 2001.

Marilyn Glenville, *Natural Solutions to Infertility: How to increase your chances of conceiving and preventing miscarriage*, Piatkus, UK, 2000.

Francesca Naish, *Natural Fertility: The complete guide to avoiding or achieving conception*, Milner, Australia, 2000 (revised edition).

Dr Miriam Stoppard, *Conception, Pregnancy and Birth,* Dorling Kindersley, UK, 2002.

Ruth Trickey and Kaz Cooke, *Women's Trouble: Natural and medical solutions,* Allen & Unwin, Australia, 2000.

Infertility treatment

Loraine Brown, *Why Me: The real-life guide to infertility*, Simon and Schuster, Australia, 1998.

Debra Fulghum Bruce and Samuel Thatcher, *Making A Baby: Everything you need to know to get pregnant*, Ballantine, USA, 2000.

Anna Furse, *Your Essential Infertility Companion: A user's guide to tests, technology and therapies*, Thorsons, HarperCollins, UK, 2001 (revised edition).

Professor Robert Jansen, *Getting Pregnant: A compassionate resource to overcoming infertility*, Allen & Unwin, Australia, 2003 (revised edition).

Resolve, The National Infertility Association, *Resolving Infertility: Understanding the options and choosing solutions when you want to have a baby,* HarperCollins, USA, 1999.

Personal stories

Linda Fiske, *The Child Within: Surviving the shattered dreams of motherhood*, Hill of Content, Australia, 2001.

Amanda Hampson, *Battle With The Baby Gods*, Transworld, Australia, 1998.

Julia Masters, *The Rollercoaster: A country couple's ride with in-vitro fertilisation*, Wakefield Press, Australia, 2000.

Hans Morse, *A Childless World: A husband's personal account of infertility*, Pan Macmillan, Australia, 2001.

Miscarriage and loss

Amanda Collinge, Sue Daniel and Heather Grace Jones, *Always A Part Of Me: Surviving childbearing loss*, ABC, Australia, 2002.

Ann Douglas and John R Sussman, *Trying Again: a guide to pregnancy after miscarriage, stillbirth and infant loss*, Taylor Publishing, USA, 2000.

Professor Lesley Regan, *Miscarriage: What every woman needs to know*,Orion, UK, 2001 (revised edition).

Adrienne Ryan, *A Silent Love: Personal stories of coming to terms with miscarriage* Penguin, Australia, 2000.

Support

Janet Balaskas, *Easy Exercises For Pregnancy*, Frances Lincoln, UK, 1997.

Kate Bourne, *Sometimes It Takes Three To Make A Baby*, Melbourne IVF, Australia, 2002 (Illustrated book for young children explaining egg donation).

Katrina Bowman and Louise Ryan, *Twins: A practical and emotional guide to parenting twins*, Allen & Unwin, Australia, 2002.

Arlene Eisenberg, Sandee E. Hathaway, Heidi E. Murkoff, *What to Eat When You're Expecting*, Workman Publishing company, USA, 1986.

Natascha Mirosch , *Going It Alone: The single women's guide to pregnancy and birth*, New Holland, Australia, 2002.

Quit, *How to Refuse The Next Cigarette*, Penguin, Australia, 2003.

Gill Thorn, *Not Too Late: Having a baby after 35*, Bantam Books, Transworld Publishers, UK, 1998.

Rosalind Widdowson, *Yoga For Pregancy*, Chancellor Press, Hamlyn, UK, 2002.

Bibliography

Brown, Lorraine, *Why Me: The real-life guide to infertility*, Simon & Schuster, Australia, 1998.

Douglas, Ann and Sussman, John R, MD, *Trying Again: A guide to pregnancy after miscarriage, stillbirth and infant loss*, Taylor Publishing Company, Dallas, USA, 2000.

Fulghum Bruce, Debra and Thatcher, Samuel, MD, PhD *Making A Baby: Everything you need to know to get pregnant*, Ballantine Books, New York, 2000.

Furse, Anna, *Your Essential Infertility Companion: A user's guide to tests, technology and therapies*, Thorsons, London, 2001.

Gardner, David K, Weissman, Ariel, Howles, Colin M, Shoham, Zeev (editors), *Textbook of Assisted Reproductive Techniques: Laboratory and clinical perspectives,* Martin Dunitz Ltd, London, 2001.

IVF Friends Inc, *Patient Letters: Personal experiences of IVF*, IVF Friends Inc., Melbourne, Australia, 1995.

Jansen, Professor Robert, *Getting Pregnant: A compassionate resource to overcoming infertility*, Allen & Unwin, Sydney, 1997.

Jansen, Professor Robert and Mortimer, David (editors), *Towards Reproductive Certainty: Fertility and genetics beyond 1999*, The Parthenon Publishing Group, London, 1999.

Oke, Kay (editor), *Taking Charge of Your Infertility*, Melbourne IVF, Australia, 1999.

Resolve, The National Infertility Association, *Resolving Infertility: Understanding the options and choosing solutions when you want to have a baby*, HarperCollins, USA, 1999.

Ryan, Adrienne, *A Silent Love: Personal stories of coming to terms with miscarriage*, Penguin Books, Australia, 2000.

Shoham, Zeev, Howles, Colin M, Jacobs, Howard S (editors), *Female Infertility Therapy: Current practice*, Martin Dunitz Ltd., London, 1999.

Index

20180871R00197

Printed in Great Britain
by Amazon